FOOD and AGRICULTURE

23. 6 80

A **SCIENTIFIC** *Book*
AMERICAN

FOOD and AGRICULTURE

W. H. FREEMAN AND COMPANY
San Francisco

The Cover

The picture on the cover symbolizes the theme of this SCIENTIFIC AMERICAN book: food and agriculture. It is a detail of a special computer-enhanced satellite image of a scene in the Imperial Valley in southern California; the dark, seemingly jagged line running diagonally across the picture is an irrigation canal along the border between the U.S. and Mexico. The image was made by researchers in the Federal Systems Division of the International Business Machines Corporation who are working under contract with the National Aeronautics and Space Administration on the development of a new digital-processing technique for generating precisely corrected false-color composite images from data obtained by the multispectral scanning system on the LANDSAT earth-resources satellites. In such false-color composites healthy vegetation is usually shown in red. Differences in patterns of land ownership and other agricultural practices are evident in this particular view, made from data obtained by LANDSAT 2 in May, 1975, from an altitude of 570 miles. A LANDSAT photograph of the entire Imperial Valley appears on page 2.

Library of Congress Cataloging in Publication Data

Main entry under title:

Food and Agriculture.

"A Scientific American book."
Articles from the September 1976 issue of Scientific American.
Bibliography: p.
Includes index.
1. Agriculture—Addresses, essays, lectures.   2. Food supply—Addresses, essays, lectures.   3. Nutrition—Addresses, essays, lectures.
I. Scientific American.
S523.F65   630   76-43064
ISBN 0-7167-0382-3
ISBN 0-7167-0381-5 pbk.

The twelve chapters in this book originally appeared as articles in the September 1976 issue of *Scientific American*.

Printed in the United States of America

9 8 7 6 5 4 3 2

Contents

Foreword

How will the world feed the three billion additional people who will join the population between now and the end of the century? That question provides the occasion for the publication of this book. It is answered by a group of authors who are otherwise occupied in making their answers work in the gardens, paddy fields, croplands and ranges of the world. Each author, from his own firsthand experience, testifies to the urgency of the problems of hunger and poverty, now exacerbated by rapid population growth. From their common experience, however, they concur in the judgement that mankind has, for the first time in history, the capability to lift these ancient curses from human life—to increase food supplies faster than population growth and, with the democratization of material well-being, to bring population growth to a halt at a number that is in reasonable balance with the finite resources of this planet.

Such a conclusion runs counter to that put abroad by authors less directly engaged in the work at hand. The misinformed popular consensus holds that the exploding populations of the poor (underdeveloped) countries have overrun their agricultural resources. The ethic of the triage and the lifeboat instructs the people of the rich (developed) countries to quarantine certain "basket case" nations in their misery and to be ready to repel "boarding parties" of the desperate poor.

In fact, the peoples of the underdeveloped countries have outgrown not their resources, but the subsistence-agriculture technology they have practiced since the dawn of history. By conservative estimates, presently demonstrated agricultural technology, if applied to all land now in cultivation, could support a world population of 45 billion. That is three or four times the number at which it is reckoned the population will stabilize, if all goes well, in the next century. In reserve are the increases in productivity that are bound to come with the application of the powerful tools of molecular biology to the genetic engineering of crop plants.

The fact that it is now technologically feasible to eliminate hunger from human experience carries immense force against the political, economic and social obstacles that stand in the way. The transfer of modern agricultural technology from the developed to the underdeveloped countries is gathering perceptible momentum. A cycle of U.N. conferences on population, food and resources has established the framework for concerted international action on a world agricultural development plan. The U.S. National Academy of Sciences is engaged in a study, under presidential directive, of ways to mobilize U.S. scientific resources for the effort.

Much of modern agricultural technology is American. As is well known, one American on the farm feeds more than 50 fellow citizens off the farm. This is the outcome of the well-placed faith in science and in education expressed by the founding of the land-grant colleges in the middle of the last century. From these institutions have come not only such feats of biological engineering as the development of high-yield strains of corn, wheat, rice and potato but well-proven techniques for moving new knowledge from the laboratory to the farm.

The chapters in this book were first published in the September 1976 issue of SCIENTIFIC AMERICAN, which was the twenty-seventh in the series of single-topic issues published annually by the magazine. The editors herewith express appreciation to their colleagues at W. H. Freeman and Company, the book-publishing affiliate of SCIENTIFIC AMERICAN, for the enterprise that has made the contents of this issue so speedily available in book form.

THE EDITORS*

September, 1976

*BOARD OF EDITORS: Gerard Piel (Publisher), Dennis Flanagan (Editor), Francis Bello (Associate Editor), Philip Morrison (Book Editor), Trudy E. Bell, Brian P. Hayes, Jonathan B. Piel, John Purcell, James T. Rogers, Armand Schwab, Jr., Jonathan B. Tucker, Joseph Wisnovsky

1

Food and Agriculture

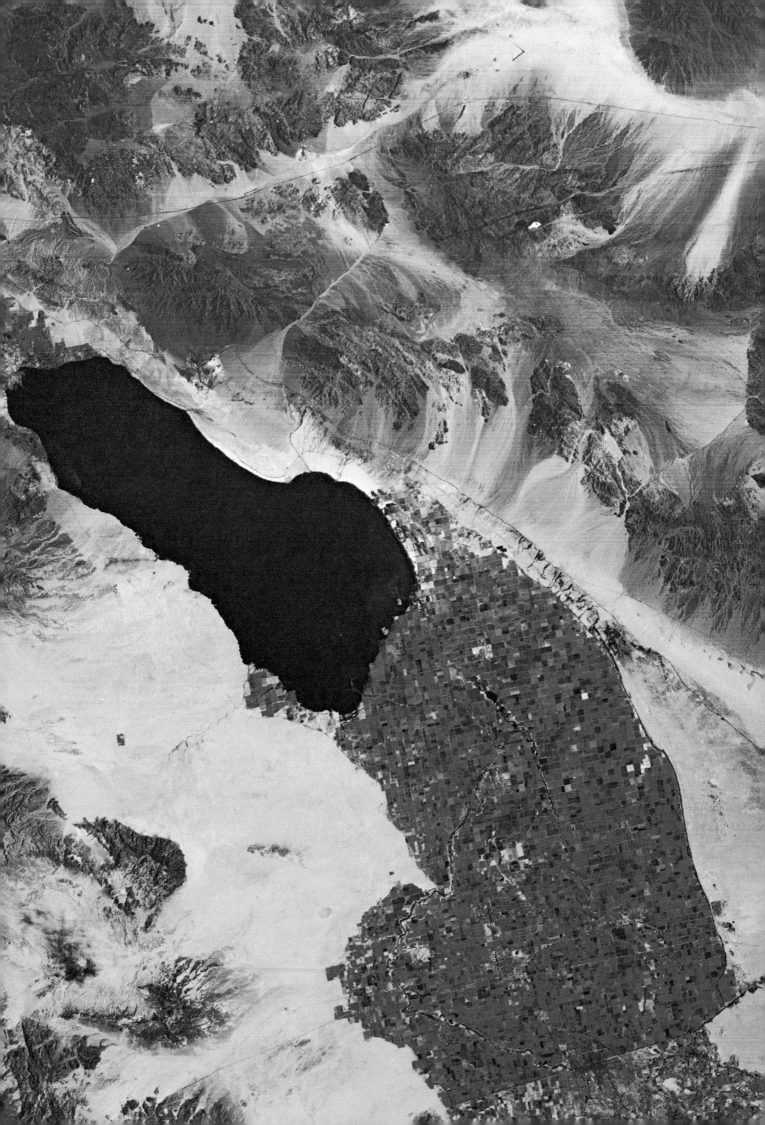

Food and Agriculture

STERLING WORTMAN

*Introducing a volume about the world food problem.
The situation is hopeful, with one proviso: that
the development efforts of agrarian countries be
concentrated less on industry and more on agriculture*

The world food situation is serious, even precarious. It is also true that the world may have, for the first time in history, the ability to deal effectively with the interacting problems of food production, rapid population growth and poverty. What, then, is the moral of this *Scientific American* book dealing with food and agriculture?

Certain facts are indisputable. The world population was two billion in 1930, reached three billion in 1960, stands today at four billion and is headed for six billion by the end of the century. On the other hand, the annual rate of increase appears now to be reaching a peak. The worldwide rate of food production has recently been increasing along with population. The "green revolution" of the late 1960's represented a significant improvement in grain-crop productivity, primarily in parts of Asia and Latin America; China now feeds its vast population; India has just reported a bumper crop of grain. Yet year in and year out much of the world cannot feed itself and has been making ends meet with food from diminishing surplus

stocks in a few countries. Hundreds of millions of people in scores of countries live in abject poverty, suffering from chronic malnutrition that reinforces their poverty and subject to calamitous famines when their precarious food supplies are reduced by drought or floods or wars [see "The Dimensions of Human Hunger," by Jean Mayer, page 14].

Faced with these facts, there are serious scholars who forecast impending starvation of major international proportions. Some, pointing out that more than enough food is being produced in many parts of the world, advocate a radical redistribution of that food from the rich countries to the poor ones. Others propose a different solution: they would abandon the populations of the countries whose prospects for survival they consider virtually nil by withholding from them food and technical and economic aid, sending selective help instead only to those countries they give a reasonable chance of survival. On the other hand, many students of the problem are optimistic that food supplies will improve gradually as scientific knowledge

and technology are widely applied to improve agricultural productivity, as population growth rates decline under the impact of mass education and family planning and also as an implicit accompaniment of economic advances.

The evidence assembled in this issue, to my mind, justifies the second of the two broad attitudes I have described, but with an important proviso: The improvement will come about only if it is actively engendered by radically new public policies both in the rich nations and in the poor nations themselves. It is important to realize that the mutual relations among the problems of low agricultural productivity, high population growth rates and poverty offer opportunity as well as difficulty. An all-out effort to increase food production in the poor, food-deficit countries may be the best means of raising incomes and accumulating the capital for economic development, and thus for moving the poor countries through the demographic transition to moderate rates of population growth.

Since 1798, when Thomas Malthus published *An Essay on the Principle of Population*, there have been repeated warnings that man's numbers, which are subject to exponential increase, could—or at some time surely would—overtake food supplies, which Malthus assumed could only increase arithmetically. Over the years there have been localized famines and some food shortages of wider extent: there were major shortages in the early 1920's following World War I, in the late 1940's and early 1950's after World War II, in the mid-1960's after two years of drought on the Indian subcontinent and most recently in 1972, when world grain production fell 35

IMPERIAL VALLEY in south-central California is the site of the largest single expanse of irrigated agriculture in the Western Hemisphere; its almost flat floor contains nearly 500,000 acres of highly productive cropland, with the major crops being barley, alfalfa, sugar beets, rye, cotton, vegetables and livestock. The main portion of the valley extends from the Salton Sea in the north to the Mexican border in the south. The average yearly rainfall here is about three inches, and the temperature usually exceeds 100 degrees Fahrenheit on more than 110 days of the year. The valley receives most of its irrigation water from the Colorado River by way of the 80-mile-long All-American Canal (*dark line at lower right*). The Salton Sea was formed between 1905 and 1907 when water was accidentally diverted from the Colorado into the dry, salt-covered depression known as the Salton Sink, which was then about 280 feet below sea level. Irrigation-drainage water from the Imperial Valley and the Coachella Valley (to the northwest) has since stabilized the saline lake against evaporation. This digitally processed false-color composite image, made from data obtained by the LANDSAT 1 earth-resources satellite on May 22, 1975, was supplied by the IBM Federal Systems Division; an enlargement of the area in the vicinity of the border between U.S. and Mexico appears on the cover of this book.

million tons and the U.S.S.R. bought heavily on the international market. Yet it was not until less than 15 years ago that people began to appreciate the serious and chronic nature of the world food problem.

It was in 1963 that Lester R. Brown, who was then working in the U.S. Department of Agriculture, published a paper in which he presented projections to the year 2000 of changes in grain production and net trade. The projections (not predictions but extrapolations of the trends then current) suggested that even though the developing countries could be tripling their grain output by 2000, exports from developed countries to less developed ones would need to be more than quadrupled to meet the ever rising demand. In a 1965 paper Brown noted that before 1940 the less developed areas of Asia, Africa and Latin America had all been net exporters of wheat, rice, corn and other grains to the more industrial nations. By the end of World War II, however, the less developed countries had lost their surplus and the net flow was reversed. The export of grain from the developed world to the less developed one rose from an average of four million tons a year in 1948 to some 25 million tons in 1964. Brown concluded: "The less developed world is losing the capacity to feed itself." Since then the flow of grain from a few developed countries to the developing regions has continued to rise; indeed, in the recently ended crop year it appears that almost all the interregional grain exports came from the U.S., Canada and Australia [*see illustration on page 9*].

If the grain-production trends of the past 15 years continue, according to the International Food Policy Research Institute, the food-grain deficit of developing countries with market economies will be about 100 million tons a year by 1985–1986. If the rather lower rate of increase in production characteristic of the past seven years prevails instead, their annual deficit could reach a staggering 200 million tons.

Those projections are specifically for the poor countries that cannot produce enough food to feed themselves. There are developing countries (Thailand and Argentina) that export food and a few, such as China, that are virtually self-sufficient in food. And there are many developed countries that need to import food and are able to pay for it; there is nothing about a localized food deficit that foreign exchange cannot cure. The problem, then, is centered in the developing countries with food deficits. The complexity of the task of improving the situation of those countries derives from their particular characteristics.

Whereas in 1974 the per capita gross national product was $6,720 in Sweden, $6,640 in the U.S., $2,770 in Italy and $2,300 in the U.S.S.R., some 90 countries had a per capita product below $500; about 40 of these had one of less than $200. These are statistical averages: in most market-economy developing countries there are sharp income disparities, and income levels among the masses of rural people are far below any average. As a group these countries have inadequate foreign-exchange reserves; many of them depend on one raw-material export or at most a few; their balance of trade is usually negative and they are heavily in debt.

Developing countries are agrarian, with from 50 to 80 percent of their people in rural areas, often far from centers of government. For most of them the source of livelihood is the production of food or fiber crops or the husbanding of animals that are adapted to local soil and climatic conditions. The productivity of their crops and their animals is in most cases abysmally low.

The ratio of land to population is dwindling; in a number of countries the amount of cultivated land per person is less than an acre. Even a few decades ago food production could be increased in most countries by bringing additional land under cultivation or extending grazing areas; now that option is disappearing in many regions. Moreover, as land has been divided repeatedly among generations of heirs, most family holdings have become extremely small.

The rural people have little access to education or health care. Housing is substandard. Life expectancy is low, and large families have traditionally provided a source of labor and of security for parents in their later years. Often out of sight and out of mind of urban-based governments, these rural populations are the poorest of the poor.

Another handicap for many of these countries is their small size: in almost 80 the population is less than five million, and in more than 30 of these it is less

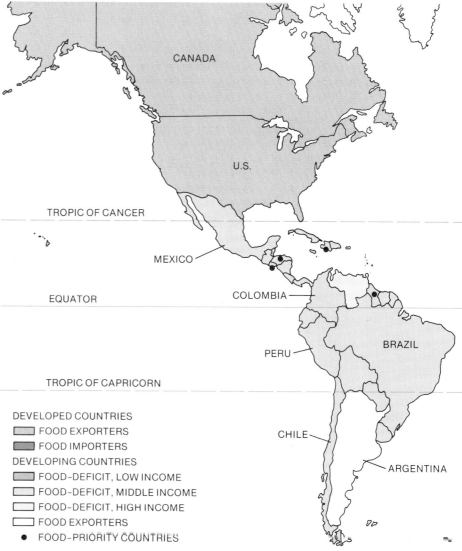

IMPACT OF FOOD DEFICITS AND POVERTY is concentrated in the broad band of developing nations, as is shown in this map based on categories established by the International Food Policy Research Institute (IFPRI). A few developed countries are major exporters of

than a million. Such nations cannot expect to develop for themselves the full range of scientific and other professional services required in fields that are important to development; they must rely on external resources. The developing countries' lack of institutions and trained personnel is exacerbated by the fact that many of them are newly independent. Of the countries listed by the United Nations as being least developed or as being "most seriously affected" by recent economic stresses, 36 have become independent since 1945, 29 of them only since 1960. The departure of the colonial powers left many of them without the skills needed to improve food-crop production, with weak institutions and in many cases without the reliable market outlets or sources of supply that had existed when they were part of a colonial system.

Moreover, as colonies their basic food crops and food animals had been neglected. Many developing countries have numerous centers for research on coffee, cacao, oil palm, rubber and jute and other cash export crops, but until a few years ago there were few such centers for wheat, rice, corn, food legumes, root crops, vegetables and other crops essential for feeding rural and urban populations. Even since independence the attention of governments and industry has tended to remain centered on estate and industrial crops that can generate foreign exchange. There has been little concern for providing the research and training and for establishing the market systems that characterized formerly successful efforts in connection with export crops. In many of these essentially agrarian countries the people in power are military officers, lawyers, businessmen, engineers or others who know little about agriculture or the science that underlies it.

Now increasing numbers of people, most of them in the countryside, are becoming restless. With advances in mass communication and in transportation these long-neglected people are becoming aware that only a small fraction of the citizenry are enjoying the comforts of life. Seeing no hope for themselves or their children, they are receptive to any ideology that offers them what they hold most important: food, clothing, housing, health care, education, security—and hope.

Accordingly government leaders are being made increasingly aware that unless they take steps to develop their rural areas they may well be faced with continuing unrest and violence and even revolution. A new political will to deal with agriculture is emerging. Trends in world food supplies have contributed to the new sense of emergency. With the dwindling of reserves of grain in the U.S. and some other food-surplus countries, many leaders of developing countries can no longer count on continuing access to the cheap (or even free) supplies that have enabled them to keep

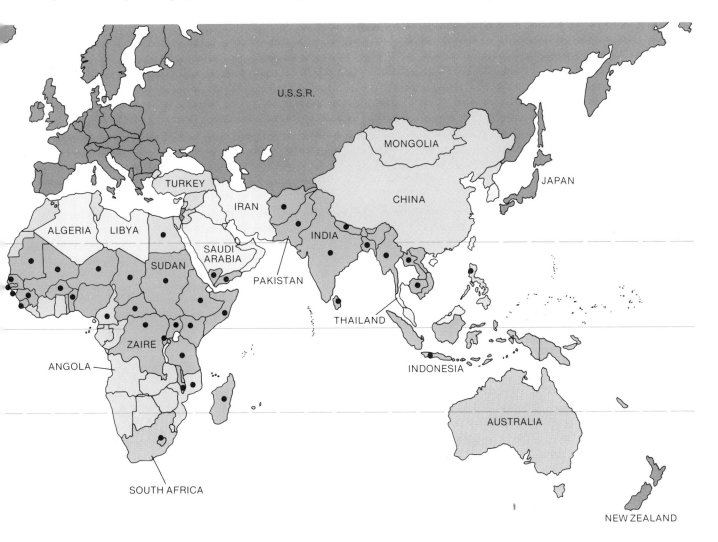

food; the rest have net food deficits but can pay to import food. Almost all developing countries have a food deficit and only those in the relatively high-income category have the foreign exchange with which to buy food without constraint. The United Nations has identified 43 "food-priority countries" (*black disks*) with especially low incomes, inadequate diets and large projected cereal-grain deficits.

food costs low in their urban areas while continuing to neglect their agricultural areas. With the high cost of food on international markets requiring large outlays of scarce foreign exchange, some governments are for the first time being compelled, for political reasons, to worry about their farm populations. The reduction of the surpluses could ironically be one of the more favorable events of recent times—if it galvanizes governments into action.

To understand the kind of action that is required it is helpful to consider the stages through which agricultural systems move and the transformations of the current century. For thousands of years men have practiced traditional subsistence agriculture. Ever since hunters and gatherers took up sedentary farming there has been a long and slow evolution of countless systems of crop and animal production, many of which persist today [see "The Plants and Animals That Nourish Man," by Jack R. Harlan, page 57]. Traditional farming systems involve only man, his animals, his seed and his land, with little need for the involvement of governments or industry or for cooperation with others. The productivity of such systems is largely limited by soil fertility and climate, and family income in cash or in kind depends in part on the size of the farm operation that can be handled with family labor. The great bulk of the world's farmers still practice some form of subsistence farming.

A significantly different kind of agricultural development has been introduced largely within this century, based on science and technology and generated mainly by consumer demand. This agricultural revolution, in which the Western nations have pioneered and excelled, has been fostered by research and educational institutions, industry and public agencies, and by the efforts of increasingly sophisticated and innovative farm populations [see "The Agriculture of the U.S.," by Earl O. Heady, page 77]. The past 75 years have seen the introduction of more efficient crop varieties and animal strains; the development, improvement and widening application of chemical fertilizers and means for controlling disease and insect pests; the introduction of ever more farm machinery and the trend toward industrialized farming and other "agribusiness," all underlain by more extensive networks of roads, electric power and communications.

What we begin to see now, and what needs to be promoted, is not simply the spread of this scientific-technical way of life to the developing countries but a new stage of deliberate, forced-pace agricultural and rural-development campaigns driven by several new forces more insistent than rising consumer demand [see "The Development of Agriculture in Developing Countries," by W. David Hopper, page 137]. Literally scores of countries are looking for ways to raise food production, incomes and living standards among the rural masses, not in the 50 or 75 years such changes required in the Western countries but in 10 or 15 years. They have no time to lose.

The first objective must be to increase food production, but more food is not enough. After all, people can get food in only three acceptable ways (if one excludes theft and violence). First, people

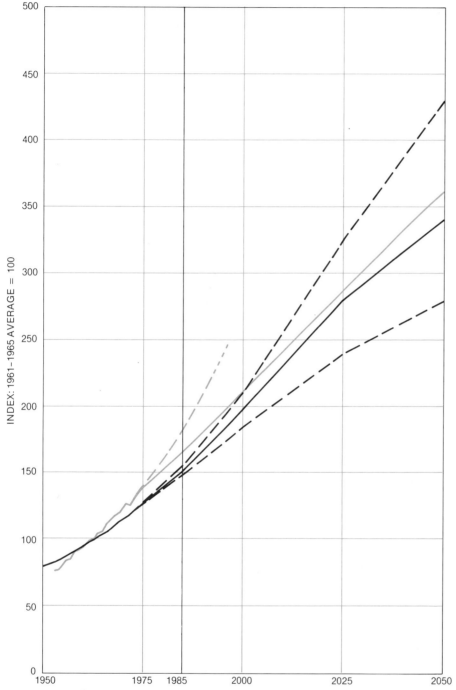

WORLDWIDE FOOD PRODUCTION seems likely to keep up with population in the near future. Here world population (*black*) and food production (*color*) are plotted as index numbers, taking the 1961–1965 averages as 100. Actual data are plotted to 1975. Thereafter three population curves are shown: the UN high, medium (*solid black*) and low projections. Two food-production projections are shown. One (*solid color*) assumes a linear rate of increase (as Malthus assumed must be the case for food production); it is based on the rate of increase (an average of three index points per year) between 1961 and 1973. Such an increase in food production lies above the medium population projection. The other food-production curve (*broken colored line*) illustrates a UN Food and Agriculture Organization projection to 1985 of the 1961–1973 rate of increase, assuming an exponential rate of growth. These curves do not imply that world food production will be adequate to meet worldwide need or even "demand."

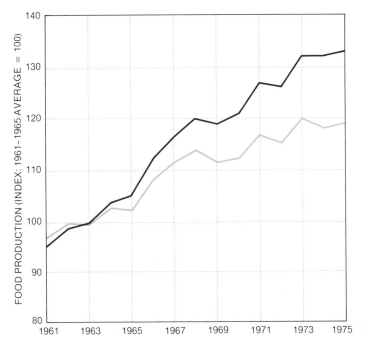
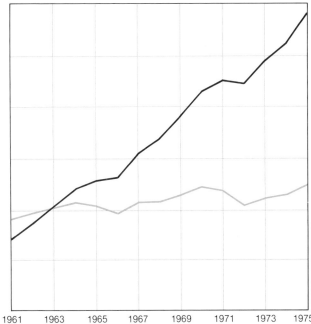

FOOD PRODUCTION has increased in developed (*left*) and developing (*right*) countries at similar rates (*black curves*). As FAO data show, however, the rise is largely nullified in developing countries, where rapid population growth reduces production per capita (*color*).

who have land may be able to grow their own food, or at least some of it for part of the year; ways must be sought to enable them to increase their output. Second, people can receive food as a gift, but that only buys important living time and is not a continuing solution to their basic poverty. Third, people can buy food if they have money, but hungry people do not have money—in the developing countries or in the U.S. or wherever else people are hungry.

Thus there are two components to the solution of the food problem: increased production of food, primarily in the developing countries, and widespread increases in family incomes, particularly among the poor. The higher incomes will have to come primarily from the increased productivity and profitability of agriculture, from the development of industry (primarily labor-intensive industries and particularly in the rural areas where most people live), from employment in construction and public works and from the generation of the diverse services that will be in demand as rural areas become more prosperous.

The bulk of the food supply of most agrarian countries is produced by individual farmers with tiny family-operated holdings. Improvement of the productivity and income of these people will require the introduction of new high-yielding, science-based crop and animal production systems tailored to the unique combination of soil, climate, biological and economic conditions of individual localities in every nation [see "Agricultural Systems," by Robert S. Loomis, page 69]. Needed now are concerted campaigns to move into the

countryside not only with knowledge of new techniques and new varieties of crops and animals but also with roads and power systems, with inputs such as fertilizers, pesticides and vaccines for animal diseases and with arrangements for credit and for marketing agricultural products.

All of this is aimed at generating the main ingredient for rural development: increased income for large numbers of farm families. Until their purchasing power is increased through on-farm or off-farm employment there can be no solution to the world food problem. Extending science-based, market-oriented production systems to the rural masses can enable the developing countries to substantially expand their domestic markets for urban industry. As farm families attain larger disposable incomes through increased agricultural profits they can become buyers of goods and services, providing more jobs and higher incomes not only on farms but also in rural trading centers and in the cities. What I am suggesting, in other words, is that the improvement of agricultural productivity is the best route to economic advancement for the agrarian developing countries.

Let me mention three nonsolutions to the problems of food and hunger that are often proposed. Larger harvests in the few remaining surplus-production countries, notably the U.S., Canada and Australia, are not a solution. Those countries do need to improve their productivity to create surpluses for export, to maintain their balance of payments and to respond when necessary to emer-

gency needs for food caused by calamities anywhere in the world. To continue to allocate free or low-cost food to governments that neglect their own rural areas, however, is counterproductive. It simply allows governments to put off the tedious and unglamorous task of helping their own people to help themselves.

The introduction into developing countries of Western-style, large-scale mechanized farming is also not a solution. Such methods may be appropriate for thinly populated areas in some countries and may help governments to get food supplies under national control quickly, but there remains the problem of getting food from large farms even to nearby individual families that have no money to pay for it. Even if the product of such farms were destined solely for urban consumers, it would deprive the smaller farmers of such markets for their own produce. Perhaps more important, most large-scale mechanized agriculture is less productive per unit area than small-scale farming can be. The farmer on a small holding can engage in intensive, high-yield "gardening" systems such as intercropping (planting more than one crop in the same field, perhaps in alternate rows), multiple cropping (planting several crops in succession, up to four a year in some places), relay planting (sowing a second crop between the rows of an earlier, maturing crop) or other techniques that require attention to individual plants. The point is that mechanized agriculture is very productive in terms of output per man-year, but it is not as productive per unit of land as the highly intensive systems are. And it is arable land that is scarce for most farmers in many countries.

Finally, the advent of synthetic foods, single-cell proteins and so on will not be a solution. These products may prove to be valuable additives, but they have to be bought before they can be eaten. The hungry have no money, and the manufacture of novel foods does not provide any increase in income for the poor. The only real solution to the world food problem is for poor countries to quickly increase the production of crops and animals—and incomes—on millions of small farms, thus stimulating economic activity.

Is there any hope that this can be done? The assertion that this is the right time for "a bold new program" is not, after all, new. It was in 1949 that President Truman proposed his Point Four technical-aid program, arguing that "for the first time in history, humanity possesses the knowledge and the skill to relieve the suffering" of the world's poor. Is it any more reasonable to call for a new initiative today than it was a quarter of a century ago? The fact is that since then there have been a number of significant and hopeful developments.

First of all, the nature of the problem has become understood only during the past dozen years or so. I remarked

above that the first projections of food requirements and deficits to the end of the century appear to have been made by Lester Brown in 1963 and 1965. The first comprehensive appraisal was undertaken in 1966 by some 125 American scientists and other specialists under the auspices of the President's Science Advisory Committee; their report titled "The World Food Problem" appeared in 1967. There have been many other reviews since then, the most recent major one being that of the World Food Conference in 1974. In the past 10 years the world has begun to mobilize to deal with technical and organizational requirements. The increased production of basic food crops on all farms everywhere has at last been accepted as the primary solution to the world food problem.

The transfer of technology in agriculture is not a simple process, however, and the second hopeful development is that its complexity is now reasonably well understood. Whereas most types of technology are widely applicable, the biological components of agricultural technology are not. They need to be tailored for each locality and developed in it.

For example, when Norman E. Borlaug of the Rockefeller Foundation began to work on wheat production in Mexico in the 1940's, he first tried to

raise the yields of local varieties by means of good management practices and the application of chemical fertilizers. The local plants simply grew very tall and leafy and were heavily attacked by rusts. He then brought in from elsewhere all the varieties he thought might possibly work in Mexico, but none of them performed under the length-of-day and climatic conditions and in the face of the locally prevalent disease organisms. Borlaug had no alternative to the slow process of breeding new wheat varieties specifically for conditions in Mexico. As he undertook the research he began to train young Mexican technicians and scientists in wheat improvement and management and to establish reliable sources of quality seed. When he had developed shorter, stiff-strawed wheat varieties resistant to disease strains prevalent in Mexico, it became possible to apply increasing amounts of fertilizers and to harvest more grain instead of more straw. The enhanced profitability of wheat production in turn induced the government and farm organizations to improve irrigation systems and the supply of necessary fertilizers and to strengthen agricultural institutions [see "The Agriculture of Mexico," by Edwin J. Wellhausen, page 87]. The point is that it was basic biological technology that was holding back advances in Mexico with wheat, as it had held

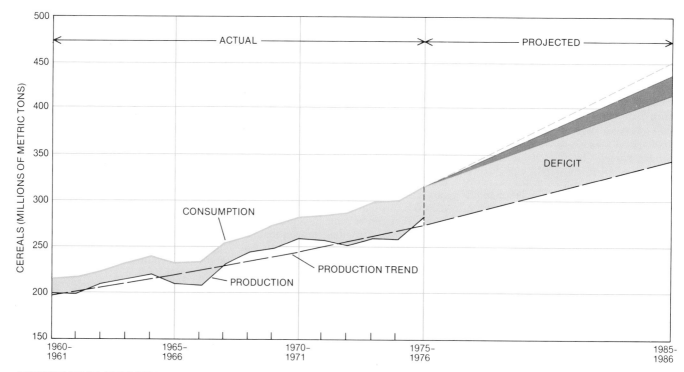

FUTURE FOOD DEFICIT in the developing countries is foreseen by IFPRI. Actual data are given, for cereal production and consumption in the market-economy developing nations that have food deficits, up to 1975–1976 (the crop year just ended). The trend of production since 1960–1961 was calculated and the trend line projected to 1985–1986. Future demand was projected from current human consumption on the basis of population growth and alternative assumptions about growth of per capita income (modified by "income elasticity" data reflecting the extent to which incremental income would be committed to cereal consumption); to this human demand, grain consumed as animal feed is added for countries rich enough to convert much grain into meat. Three demand projections are shown (*color*). One assumes no improvement in per capita consumption over the 1969–1971 level (*solid line*), one assumes low growth of income (*broken line*) and one assumes high income growth (*dotted line*). The curves measure economic demand, not actual need.

them back in Southeast Asia with rice and as it still is today in many areas of the world with many crops and animals.

The great void of food-crop and animal research in tropical and subtropical areas has now been partly filled by the establishment of 10 agricultural research and training centers in Asia, Africa and Latin America, six of them since 1970. Their work is now financed by a consortium of international agencies, national governments and a few foundations, whose support has grown from $15 million in 1972 to $65 million in 1976. Meanwhile several national governments, including those of Brazil, India, the Philippines and Pakistan, are greatly intensifying their own research efforts. For the first time in history the generation of the needed biological components of highly productive tropical agricultural systems is underway.

A third hopeful factor is that the potential for raising yields is great. As of 1971–1973 there were 135 nations in which corn was produced in significant amounts. The highest national average yield in the world was 7.2 metric tons per hectare in New Zealand; in the U.S. it was about 5.8 tons. Yet there were 112 countries with national-average yields of less than three tons, 81 of them with less than 1.5 tons! Yields of other basic food crops and animals are similarly low, reflecting the impoverishment of soils from decades if not centuries of continuous use, the failure to control diseases and pests, the low production potentials of native crop varieties and animal strains, the lack of needed nutrients in fertilizers or feed supplements and other factors.

In many of the poorer countries the application of chemical fertilizers (a good indicator of the degree of intensification of agriculture) is only beginning to spread to the basic food crops. When fertilization is combined with high-yielding varieties and improved cropping practices, yields can climb quickly and substantially, as was demonstrated beginning in the mid-1960's with wheat in India [see "The Agriculture of India," by John W. Mellor, page 101]. Of particular importance has been the creation of short, stiff-straw varieties of wheat and rice, called semidwarfs. Such varieties can utilize higher applications of nitrogen and other nutrients for the production of grain more efficiently than typical native varieties, which tend to grow excessively tall when they are heavily fertilized and to "lodge," or fall over, well before harvesting, reducing yields. For similar reasons plant height has been shortened and stalks stiffened in other grains, including corn, sorghum and barley. When high-yielding varieties are grown as dense populations, with an adequate supply of nutrients

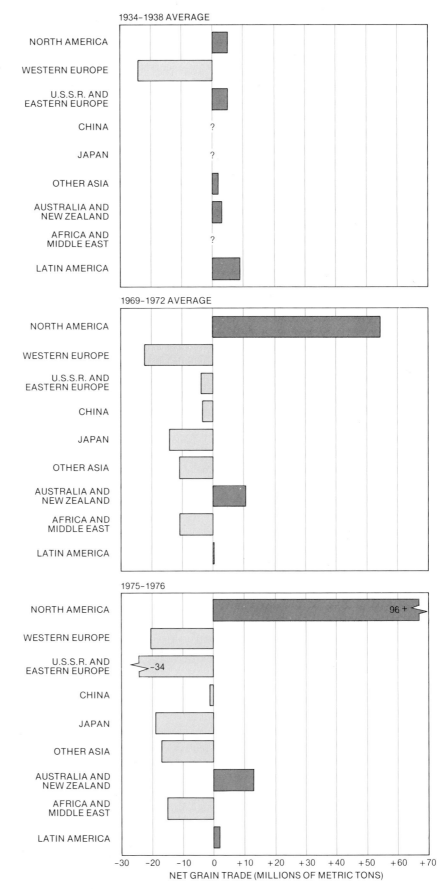

WORLD'S INCREASING DEPENDENCE on grain exports of a few countries is shown by this comparison of the trade pattern before World War II with the situation more recently and estimated figures for the past year. Data are from Lester R. Brown, the Department of Agriculture and IFPRI. Before the war most regions exported grain (*gray bars*); Western Europe imported it (*color*). Now U.S. and Canada supply most of the grain to make up deficits.

and moisture, expenditures to control diseases and insect pests often pay off handsomely, whereas at the lower-yield levels of traditional agriculture they would not. These new varieties have been the catalysts of the agricultural revolution [see "The Amplification of Agricultural Production," by Peter R. Jennings, page 125]. Higher yields result, however, when such varieties are grown in combination with fertilization, disease and pest control, higher-density planting and other measures.

A fourth new element is the availability for the first time of chemical fertilizers in sufficient quantity for widespread basic food-crop production in the developing countries. At the turn of the century the total world output of chemical nutrients was only about two million tons per year. It crept up to about 7.5 million tons by the end of World War II. Then, from 1945 to 1955, production tripled to 22 million tons. In the next decade it doubled again, and now it is appoaching 80 million tons per year. Chemical fertilizers generally can be utilized only in market-oriented systems in which a portion of the harvest is sold to cover the cost of the purchased inputs. Once limited to the production of luxury, high-value cash crops, the application of fertilizers was extended first to grain crops in the U.S. and Europe. We now understand that the green revolution was simply a significant extension of the agricultural revolution that had begun in the industrialized countries.

Fifth, it has been demonstrated that governments can take effective action if the will exists, and that many farmers will adopt new technology given reasonable opportunities to do so. When India in the 1960's successfully introduced high-yielding crop varieties, fertilizers and management practices on some 13 million hectares in five years, it demonstrated that given the availability of technology a government can increase agricultural productivity rapidly if it wants to, and that farmers will accept more productive and profitable systems if they can. There have been subsequent, less dramatic successes in Pakistan, Algeria, the Philippines, Malaysia and elsewhere. It is only in recent years that there has been evidence that small farmers as well as those with larger landholdings can be benefited if scientific and organizational efforts are genuinely directed to their particular needs. Such efforts did not begin on a substantial scale until the late 1960's.

Sixth, there is now in operation a functioning network of financial institutions, including the World Bank, the Inter-American Development Bank, the Asian Development Bank, the African Development Bank and a number of Common Market banks, as well as national agricultural banks in many of the poorer countries. During the past three or four years most major financial institutions have substantially increased their emphasis on agricultural and rural development. The world now has in operation most of the institutions needed to finance major agricultural efforts. Most of these institutions did not exist in President Truman's time; the few that were established then had limited funds and their early emphasis generally was on industrial development rather than agricultural.

Seventh, an impressive (but still inadequate) array of institutions has emerged to assist developing countries with the technical and managerial development of national programs, in some cases also offering financial aid for worthy projects and programs. Among them, in addition to the UN Food and Agriculture Organization, are agencies for bilateral aid in 16 or more industrialized nations and the staffs of the World Bank and regional banks. The Ford, Kellogg and Rockefeller foundations have active programs. Canada's International Development Research Centre has become a leading force. A new, private professional-assistance organization, the International Agricultural Development Service, began operations in 1975. Additional sources of assistance are supported by industry.

Of particular importance is the freedom, only recently gained, of some national agencies to support work aimed directly at increasing the production of basic food crops. The U.S. Agency for International Development, for example, was constrained politically until 1969 (as was Canada's comparable agency) by reluctance to become involved in direct, visible efforts abroad to increase productivity of the basic food crops, particularly the cereal grains. There was a general belief both in and out of government that other nations should not be encouraged to increase production of those crops for fear of competition with U.S. efforts to sell its surplus stocks or even give them away! For example, it was not until the last week of President Johnson's administration that the AID undertook to provide financial support for the International Rice Research Institute in the Philippines and the International Maize and Wheat Improvement Center in Mexico.

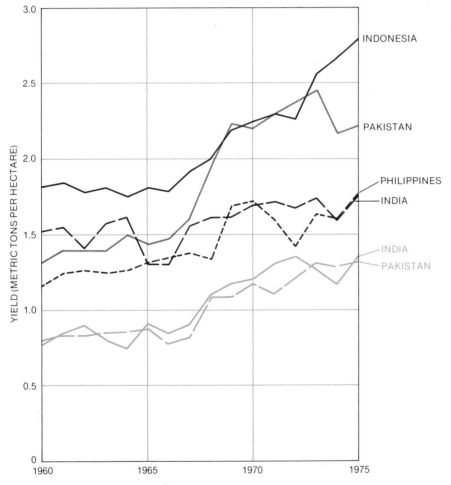

UPWARD TREND of yields of rice (*black*) and wheat (*color*) in several Asian "green revolution" countries is due primarily to introduction of high-yielding varieties, more fertilization and better farming practices. Year-by-year fluctuations are caused by weather variations.

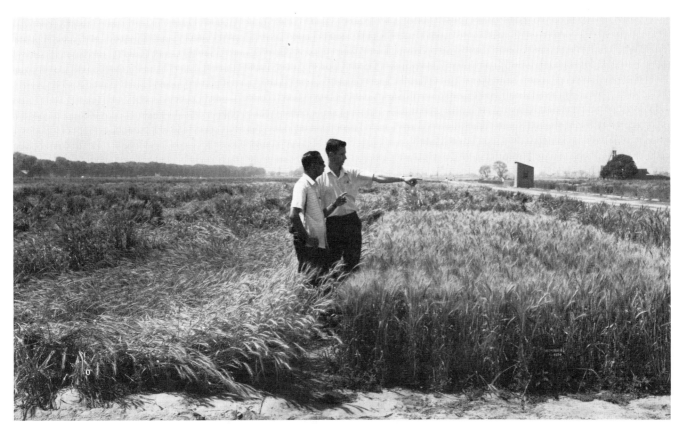

TWO WHEAT VARIETIES grow side by side in a field at the Indian Agricultural Research Institute near New Delhi. The plants at left have "lodged": having been heavily fertilized, they have grown too tall, and the stalks have bent over so that some ears of grain will break off and others may be damaged. The plants at the right have not lodged; they are newly developed varieties that have three genes for dwarfism. Resistance to lodging is critical because it makes possible the heavy fertilization that results in higher yields per hectare.

By that time it had become apparent that mounting deficits in the developing countries would soon exceed the production capacity of the U.S. and the few remaining surplus producers, and it was becoming clear that much of the hope for expanding international markets of all types rested on improving the economic position of many agrarian countries. That the U.S. and Canadian agencies were not able directly and openly to help other nations increase their basic food-crop production gave them a late start on the problem—a mere seven years ago. The handicap has since been overcome, and the agencies have responded with improved effectiveness.

Another important handicap remains. Most European and North American institutions and individuals have had little opportunity to gain experience in organizing deliberate campaigns for agricultural development. That is understandable. For many of the past 20 or 30 years the U.S. and Canada have had problems of surplus production; there has been no need for public agencies or universities to become involved in campaigns at home to raise agricultural production. Moreover, these countries have an abundance of farm entrepreneurs who are researchers and innovators in their own right, who seek out the products of research laboratories and experi-

ment stations and put them together into highly productive systems at the individual farm level. Such well-educated and exceptionally skilled farm entrepreneurs are scarce in most of the developing countries. Those who provide technical assistance will need to devise agricultural and rural-development systems for large numbers of people who are intelligent but uneducated, and who are therefore unable to undertake on their own the innovation required at the farm level.

Eighth, some governments of low-income countries are showing a new determination to develop their rural areas, with emphasis on the increased production of basic food commodities, the promotion of labor-intensive industry in rural areas and the extension of input supplies and marketing channels into areas where none have existed before.

Finally, there still remain considerable amounts of arable but currently uncultivated land that can be brought into production, except perhaps in Europe and parts of Asia [see "The Resources Available for Agriculture," by Roger Revelle, page 113].

Well-organized campaigns are needed now to force the pace of agricultural development at a rate with which few nations anywhere have had

any experience. The key elements in such campaigns are inputs of biological technology and of capital for building the infrastructure to support rural development. I have emphasized that the poor countries must do much for themselves, but they need massive help from the affluent world. For us in the U.S. that calls for a much more serious effort to direct scientific knowledge and technical skills, as well as money, specifically toward foreign rural-assistance programs.

Clearly more is at stake than the alleviation of world hunger, crucial as that is. Improving productivity in developing countries can provide millions of people not only with food but also with housing, clothing, health care, education—and hope. Enhanced agricultural productivity is the best lever for economic development and social progress in the developing world, and it is clear enough that without such development and progress there can be no long-term assurance of increased well-being or of peace anywhere in the world. The existence of new technological, financial and organizational capabilities offers a magnificent opportunity, although perhaps a fleeting one, to take effective action. The crucial question is whether or not governments will have the wisdom to act.

2

The Dimensions of
Human Hunger

The Dimensions of Human Hunger

JEAN MAYER

The number of people who are poorly nourished or undernourished can only be roughly estimated, but they probably represent an eighth of the human population. Most of them are found in Asia and Africa

Famine, fearsome and devastating though it is, can at least be attacked straightforwardly. A famine occurs in a definable area and has a finite duration; as long as food is available somewhere, relief agencies can undertake to deal with the crisis. Malnutrition, on the other hand, afflicts a far larger proportion of mankind than any famine but is harder to define and attack. Only someone professionally familiar with nutritional disease can accurately diagnose malnutrition and assess its severity. Malnutrition is a chronic condition that seems to many observers to be getting worse in certain areas. In one form or another it affects human populations all over the world, and its treatment involves not mobilization to combat a crisis but long-term actions taken to prevent a crisis—actions that affect economic and social policies as well as nutritional and agricultural ones. In the background always is the concern that too rapid an increase in population, combined with failure to keep pace in food production, will give rise to massive famines that cannot be combated.

The statistics with which the public is bombarded are of little help. What is the layman to make of statements that a billion people suffered from hunger and malnutrition last year, that 10 million children the world over are so seriously malnourished that their lives are at risk, that 400 million people live on the edge of starvation, that 12,000 people die of hunger each day and that in India alone one million children die each year from malnutrition? If the world's food problem is to be brought under control, and I believe it can be, we must first draw conceptual boundaries around it and place it in a time frame as we would a famine.

First, then, just what is the chronic hunger of malnutrition and how widespread is it? The first part of the question can be answered with assurance; the second, in spite of the statistics cited in the preceding paragraph, is really a matter of informed guesswork.

Malnutrition may come about in one of four ways. A person may simply not get enough food, which is undernutrition. His diet may lack one essential nutrient or more, which gives rise to deficiency diseases such as pellagra, scurvy, rickets and the anemia of pregnancy due to a deficiency of folic acid. He may have a condition or an illness, either genetic or environmental in origin, that prevents him from digesting his food properly or from absorbing some of its constituents, which is secondary malnutrition. Finally, he may be taking in too many calories or consuming an excess of one component or more of a reasonable diet; this condition is overnutrition. Malnutrition in this sense is a disease of affluent people in both the rich and the poor nations. In countries such as the U.S. diets high in calories, saturated fats, salt and sugar, low in fruits and vegetables and distorted toward heavily processed foods contribute to the high incidence of obesity, diabetes, hypertension and atherosclerotic disease and to marginal deficiencies of certain minerals and B vitamins. Bizarre reducing diets, which exclude entire categories of useful foods, are self-inflicted examples of the first two causes of malnutrition. The nutritional diseases of the affluent are not, however, the subject of this article. In areas where the food supply is limited the first three causes of malnutrition are often found in some combination.

In children a chronic deficiency of calories causes listlessness, muscle wastage and failure to grow. In adults it leads to a loss of weight and a reduced inclination toward and capacity for activity. Undernourished people of all ages are more vulnerable to infection and other illness and recover more slowly and with much greater difficulty. Children with a chronic protein deficiency grow more slowly and are small for their age; in severe deficiency growth stops altogether and the child shows characteristic symptoms: a skin rash and discoloration, edema and a change in hair color to an orange-reddish tinge that is particularly striking in children whose hair would normally be dark. The spectrum of protein-calorie malnutrition (PCM, as it is known to workers in the field) varies from a diet that is relatively high in calories and deficient in protein (manifested in the syndrome known as kwashiorkor) to one that is low in both calories and protein (manifested in marasmus).

Although protein-calorie malnutrition is the most prevalent form of undernourishment, diseases caused by deficiencies of specific vitamins or minerals are also widespread. It is true that the prevalence of certain classic deficiency diseases has decreased drastically since World War II. Beriberi is now rare and pellagra has been essentially eradicated, at least in its acute form; rickets is seen mostly in its adult form (osteomalacia) in Moslem women whose secluded way of life keeps them out of the sun, and scurvy is unlikely to be seen except in prisoners who are not provided with enough vitamin C. In contrast, blindness caused by the lack of vitamin A occurs with particular frequency in India, Indonesia, Bangladesh, Vietnam, the Philippines, Central America, the northeast of Brazil and parts of Africa. In remote inland areas (central Africa, the mountainous regions of South America and

POOR ALABAMA FARM FAMILY OF 1936 was photographed by Walker Evans for the Farm Security Administration of the Department of Agriculture. The farmer was Bud Fields, who lived in Hale County, in the west-central part of the state. In the intervening 40 years much of the poverty in the area has been eliminated by development programs such as the Tennessee Valley Authority. Here, as in areas of developing countries where hunger is endemic today, effects of malnutrition were severest among pregnant women and growing children.

the Himalayas) goiter, the enlargement of the thyroid resulting from a deficiency of iodine, is common. The World Health Organization estimates that up to 5 percent of such populations are afflicted with cretinism, the irreversible condition caused by iodine deficiency in the mother before or during pregnancy. From 5 to 17 percent of the men and from 10 to 50 percent of the women in countries of South America, Africa and Asia have been estimated to have iron-deficiency anemia.

The human beings most vulnerable to the ravages of malnutrition are infants, children up to the age of five or six and pregnant and lactating women. For the infant protein in particular is necessary during fetal development for the generation and growth of bones, muscles and organs. The child of a malnourished mother is more likely to be born prematurely or small and is at greater risk of death or of permanent neurological and mental dysfunction. Brain development begins *in utero* and is complete at an

early age (under two). Malnutrition during this period when neurons and neuronal connections are being formed may be the cause of mental retardation that cannot be remedied by later corrective measures. The long-term consequences, not only for the individual but also for the society and the economy, need no elaboration.

Growing children, pound for pound, require more nutrients than adults do. A malnourished child is more susceptible to the common childhood diseases, and illness in turn makes extra demands on nutritional reserves. In addition many societies, still believing the old adage about starving a fever, withdraw nourishing foods from the child just when he needs them most, thus often pushing him over the borderline into severe malnutrition. So common is the cycle of malnutrition, infection, severe malnutrition, recurrent infection and eventual death at an early age that the death rate for children up to four years old in general, and the infant mortality rate in par-

ticular, serve as one index of the nutritional status of a population as a whole. For infants less than a year old the death rate is about 250 per 1,000 births in Zambia and Bolivia, 140 in India and Pakistan and 95 in Brazil (for all its soaring gross national product). The rate in Sweden is 12 per 1,000 births; in the U.S. the average is 19, but in the country's affluent suburbs the rate equals Sweden's, whereas it rises to about 25 in the poor areas of the inner cities and as high as 60 for the most poverty-stricken and neglected members of the society: the migrant farm workers.

How reliable the figures for the developing nations are, however, is another matter. In most instances statistical reporting is as underdeveloped as the rest of the economy. Deaths, particularly of one-day-old infants, often go unreported. In all probability the rates are higher than the ones I have cited.

More precise nutritional assessments

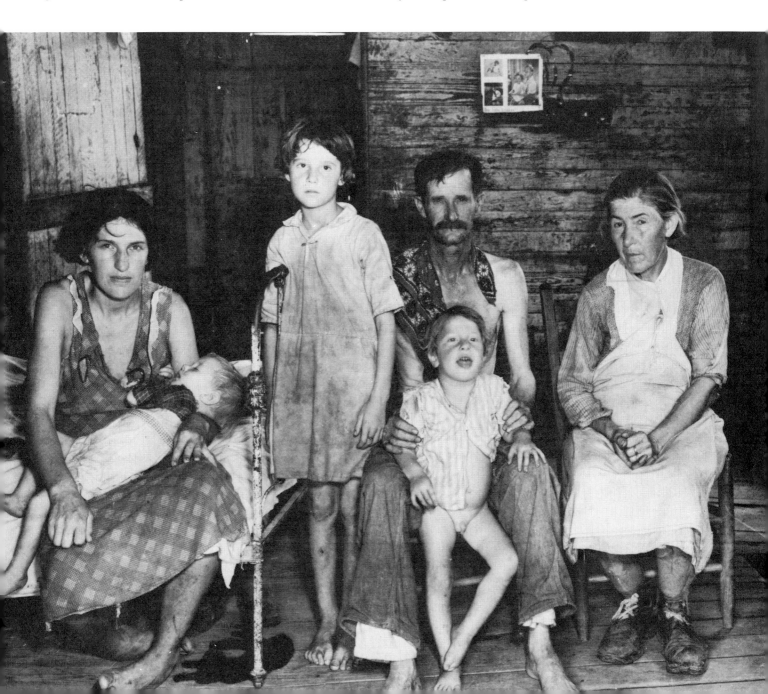

are attempted in two ways. One is to construct a "food balance sheet," which puts agricultural output, stocks and purchases on the supply side and balances them against the food used for seed for the next year's crop, animal feed and wastage and hence derives an estimate of the food that is left for human consumption. That amount can then be matched against the United Nations Food and Agriculture Organization's tables of nutritional requirements to obtain an estimate of the adequacy of the national diet.

This method has a number of drawbacks. For several reasons it tends to result in underestimates. One is that it is difficult to estimate the agricultural production in developing countries with any degree of accuracy. Farmers have every incentive to underestimate their

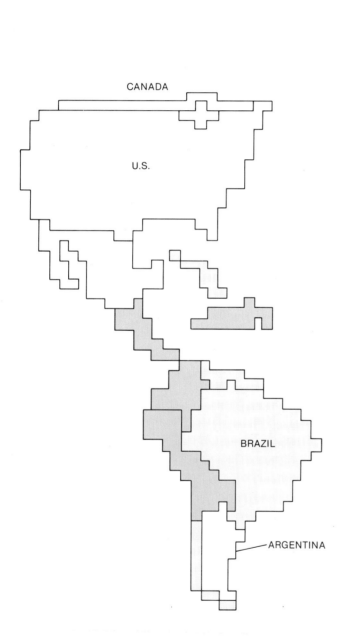

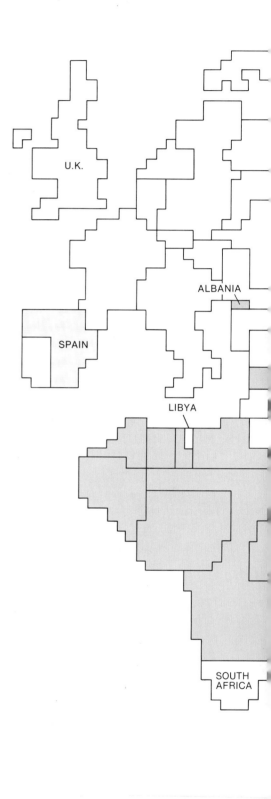

LEVEL OF ENERGY obtained from food is portrayed on a map where the area of each nation is proportional to its population. Canada, for example, occupies a large area but has a relatively small population, whereas Japan has a large population in a relatively small area. The level of energy intake is indicated by the presence or absence of color. In the countries shown in dark color the average calo-

crop: they may be able to reduce taxes and the obligatory payment of crops (often as much as 60 percent of the harvest) in rent to the landlord. Second, the foods included in the balance sheet tend to be the items that figure prominently in channels of trade: grain, soybeans and large livestock. Other farm products—eggs, small animals, fruits and vegetables—vital to a good diet but grown for family consumption or sold locally are almost impossible to count and so are ignored.

On the other hand, the balance-sheet method has certain tendencies toward overestimates. For example, it is extremely difficult to estimate the postharvest loss of crops to insects, rodents and microorganisms. The loss is known to be close to 10 percent for the U.S. wheat crop and is probably higher for other

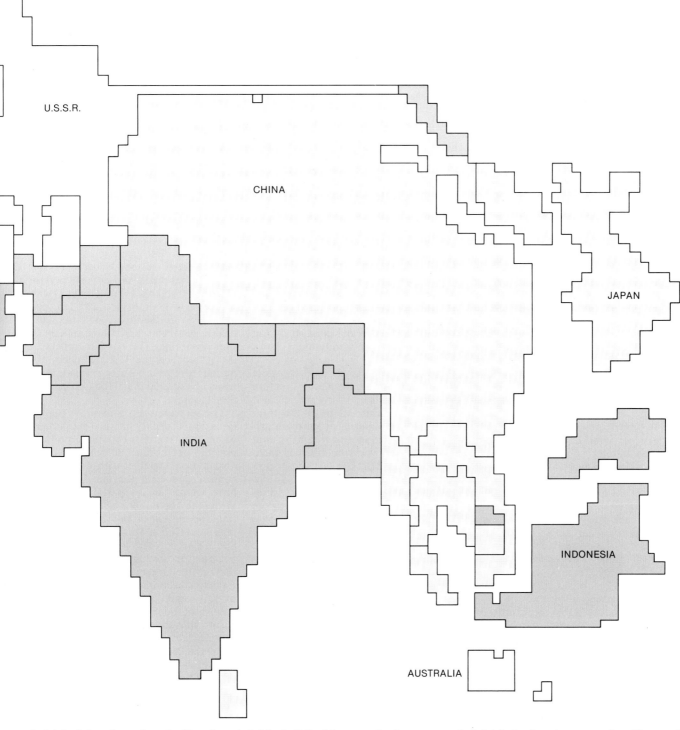

rie intake is less than adequate. (An adequate intake is defined by United Nations agencies as being about 3,000 calories per day for a man and 2,200 for a woman.) In the countries indicated by the light color the average calorie intake is adequate or as much as 10 percent above adequate, and in the countries represented in white the average calorie level is higher than adequate by at least 10 percent.

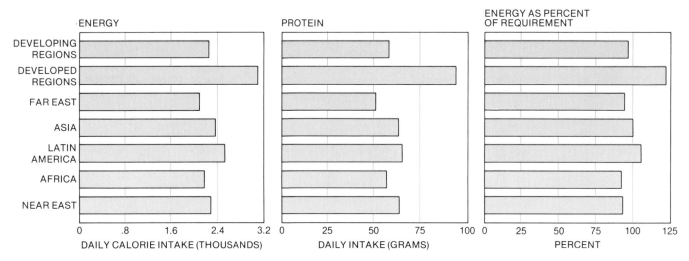

AVAILABILITY OF CALORIES AND PROTEIN is portrayed for the developed and developing regions and for several specific developing regions. The figures reflect the average daily diet per person in the various regions and are based on data assembled by the International Task Force on Child Nutrition for the UN Children's Fund. The figures for Asia refer to the centrally planned economies.

crops, even with the advanced technology available. In some tropical countries the loss can run as high as 40 percent. For all these reasons figures on food production do not provide a particularly accurate index of the amount of food actually available for consumption or the types of food actually consumed, and they make no attempt to differentiate patterns of consumption within a population. They do, however, provide rough estimates of the state of nutrition by regions [*see illustration on preceding two pages*].

The second way of estimating the degree of malnutrition within an area is to extrapolate from data compiled from hospital records and cross-sectional surveys. Statistics on illness, however, tend to be as unreliable as mortality statistics. The criteria for admission to a hospital on the basis of malnutrition vary from country to country; the records from rural areas may be sparse; the poor, among whom malnutrition and its related conditions are most likely to be found, are the least likely segment of the population to seek medical help, and if they do seek such help, the condition may then be so far advanced that the diseases associated with malnutrition, such as infantile diarrhea and pneumonia, may claim all the physician's attention, so that he misses or ignores the underlying cause.

Projections based on the results of 77 studies of nutritional status made among more than 200,000 preschool children in 45 countries of Asia, Africa and Latin America place the total number of children suffering from some degree of protein-calorie malnutrition at 98.4 million. Percentages ranged from 5 to 37 in Latin America, from 7 to 73 in Africa and from 15 to 80 in Asia (excluding China). These surveys, however, did not employ standardized proce-

dures. In some of them clinical assessments were made and in others the children were measured against international weight tables. Thus, although the general indications of such studies are useful, figures derived from them are rough at best. In order to assign reliable figures to the degree of hunger and malnutrition in the world today we would need large-scale surveys that included both clinical examinations based on an established definition of malnutrition and individual consumption surveys that determine the amount and types of food eaten and the distribution of food within each family unit.

Even if the figures derived by these methods are doubtful, the situation they reflect is clear. In my judgment it would seem reasonable to set the number of people suffering from malnutrition at 500 million and to add to that another billion who would benefit from a more varied diet. The largest concentration of such people is in Asia, Southeast Asia and sub-Saharan Africa. Clinical surveys and hospital records indicate that malnutrition wherever it exists is severest among infants, preschool children and pregnant and lactating women; that it is most prevalent in depressed rural areas and the slums of great cities; that the problem is lack of calories as much as lack of protein; that (except in areas where the people subsist largely on manioc or bananas) where calories are adequate protein tends to be adequate too, and that although a lack of food is the ultimate factor in malnutrition, that lack results from a number of causes, operating alone or in combination. A nation may lack both self-sufficiency in food production and the money to buy food or to provide the farm inputs necessary to increase production; the poorer members of the population

may lack income to buy the food that is available, and regional factors, such as customs in child-feeding and restrictions on the movement of supplies, may prevent the food from getting to the people who need it most.

On the basis of these findings one can divide the nations of the world into five groups. The first group consists of the industrialized nations, where food is plentiful but pockets of poverty persist. Here governments are able to deal with problems of malnutrition through food assistance to the poor, nutrition and health programs and nutrition-education programs. The chief members of the group are the U.S., Canada, the nations of Western Europe, Japan, Australia, New Zealand, Hong Kong and Singapore.

The second group consists of the nations with centrally planned economies, where whatever the economic philosophy the egalitarian pattern of income distribution together with government control of food supplies and distribution have seemed in the past few years to insure the populations against malnutrition due to hunger. In this category are mainland China, Taiwan, North Korea, South Korea, North Vietnam and South Vietnam. In the third group are the nations of the Organization of Petroleum Exporting Countries (OPEC), whose overall wealth is undeniable but whose pattern of income distribution does not ensure that this wealth will benefit the poor. Fourth is a group of countries in Asia, the Near East, Central America and South America that are already self-sufficient or almost self-sufficient in food production at their present level of demand. The demand, however, is impeded by an uneven distribution of income that is reflected in malnutrition in large segments of the population. Brazil, for example, has the highest economic growth rate in the world, but malnutrition is rampant in the northeast and widespread in the shantytowns surrounding the large cities.

The fifth group includes the nations the UN designates as "least developed." They have too few economic resources to provide for the people in the lowest income groups. Many of the countries are exposed to recurring droughts, floods or cyclones; some are ravaged by war. All 25 of the least developed nations are poor in natural resources and investment capital.

Looking back today, it seems incredible that in 1972 it appeared the world might soon, for the first time, be assured of an abundant food supply. The new wheat varieties of the "green revolution" had taken hold in Mexico and northwestern India, and the new varieties of rice developed in the Philippines promised a high-yield staple crop for the peoples of Southeast Asia. The harvest from the seas was still rising spectacularly (from 21 million metric tons in 1950 to 70 million in 1970—a steady increase of about 5 percent per year, outstripping the world's annual population increase of 2 percent). The worldwide production of grain was rising by an average of 2.8 percent per year, and there were substantial reserves in the form of carry-over stocks held by the principal exporting countries and of cropland held idle in the U.S. under the soil-bank program. The prospect was so rosy that the FAO suggested in 1969 that the food problems of the future might be those of surplus rather than shortage.

Although two sudden and short-term simultaneous crop failures in a number of areas and the sharp rise in oil prices were the immediate cause of the food crisis of 1972–1974, it has since become clear that four long-term factors that had been building up quietly for a long time were in any case about to alter the hopeful situation permanently. (The first short-term reversal, a reduction of crops in several parts of the world because of unfavorable weather in 1972, gave rise to a second: the massive purchases of grain by the U.S.S.R. that eliminated American reserves and caused the international prices of wheat, corn and rice to rise sharply. Moreover, the increase in oil prices effectively put the green revolution out of the reach of such countries as India, Pakistan and Bangladesh, which are poor in petroleum and other resources and have gone about as far as they can in increasing yields with traditional methods of farming. The increase in oil prices also dislocated the economies of the wealthy nations, reducing their contributions to international aid.)

Even though the situation is less serious now than it was in 1974, it is more

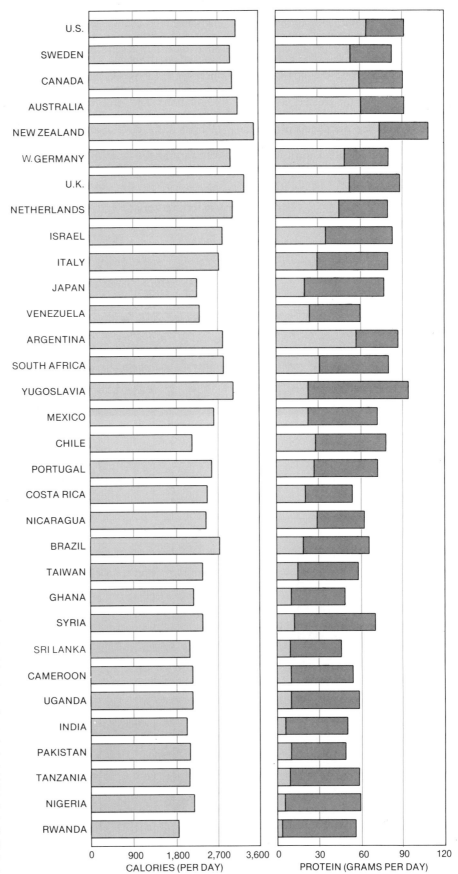

NUTRITION AND NATIONAL ECONOMY are compared in a chart that lists countries according to their gross national product as apportioned on a per capita basis. The bars at the left show the average daily calorie intake of the people in each country. In the bars at the right the full length of the bar represents the average daily protein intake of each person in grams per day, and the colored portion of the bar indicates how much of that intake is animal protein.

precarious as a result of the long-term factors. The primary long-term factor is the growth of the human population: 80 million people per year, the equivalent of the population of the U.S. every 30 months. Moreover, the population is growing most rapidly in the areas that are experiencing the greatest nutritional difficulties.

In considering the effects of population growth, however, one must bear in mind the phenomenon known as the demographic transition. It is the process whereby societies move from a stage of high birth and death rates to one of low birth and death rates. Usually the decline in death rates precedes the decline in birth rates by from one generation to three generations. On both sides of the transition the result is a stable level of population. The developed countries have made the transition or are well along in it; the developing countries are now making the transition but have traveled varying distances through it.

Alongside the inequality in population growth as a long-term factor affecting the food supply is an even greater inequality in the patterns of producing and utilizing food. It appears to be historically inevitable that as people or societies become wealthier their consumption of animal products increases. This means that more of their basic foodstuffs (grains, legumes and even fish) that could feed human beings directly are instead fed to domesticated animals such as cattle and chickens. The efficiency of the conversion of plant food into

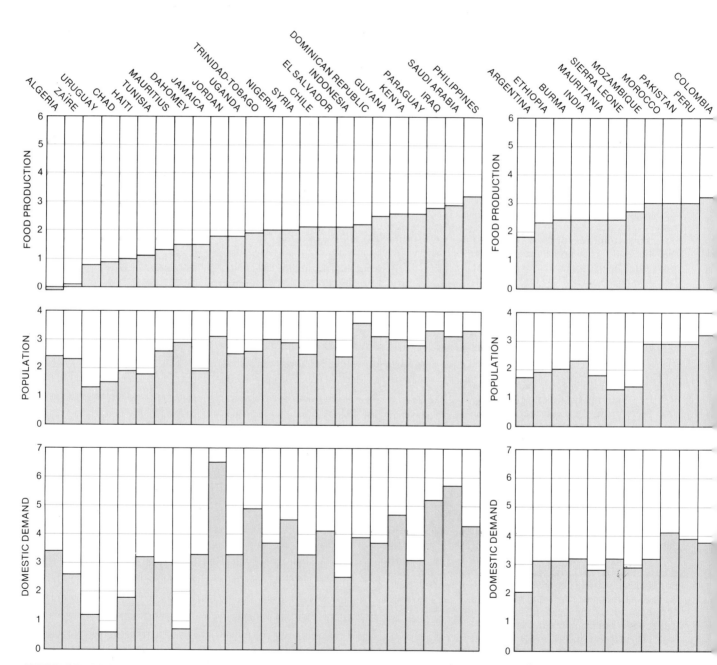

PRODUCTION FAILED TO EQUAL POPULATION GROWTH

PRODUCTION GROWTH FAILED TO EQUAL GROWTH OF DOMESTIC DEMAND

TRENDS IN FOOD PRODUCTION are traced for 71 developing countries on the basis of how each country's average annual change in food production (an increase for every country except Algeria) compares with the country's change in population and in domestic demand for food, a category that reflects not only increases in population but also the economic status of the people and their changes in preferences for food, as in a tendency to eat more meat. Each bar reflects an average annual percentage change for the period from 1953

animal food varies with the animal product but is in no case higher than the level of about 25 percent attained in milk and eggs.

The net effect of this trend is that rich countries consume far more food per capita than poor ones. For example, it has been estimated that in China each person is adequately fed on 450 pounds of grain per year; 350 pounds are consumed directly as cereal or cereal products and 100 pounds are fed to domesticated animals. In the U.S. the average

individual consumes more than 2,000 pounds of grains per year; 150 pounds are eaten directly (as bread, pasta, breakfast cereal and the like) and the rest, more than 90 percent of the total, is fed to animals.

The third source of pressure on the world's food supply has been the diminishing effectiveness of the fishing industry, an important source of protein for many poor nations. In 1970 and 1971 the total catch remained steady at

about 70 million tons. It dropped abruptly in 1972 to less than 55 million tons. The reasons for the decline are overfishing and pollution.

Finally, it has become apparent that the "miracle" of the green revolution requires more time, more work and more capital than was thought in the first flush of enthusiasm. I shall not elaborate on this point, since the green revolution is discussed in other articles in this issue. In sum, the situation as it exists today is precarious but manageable, barring

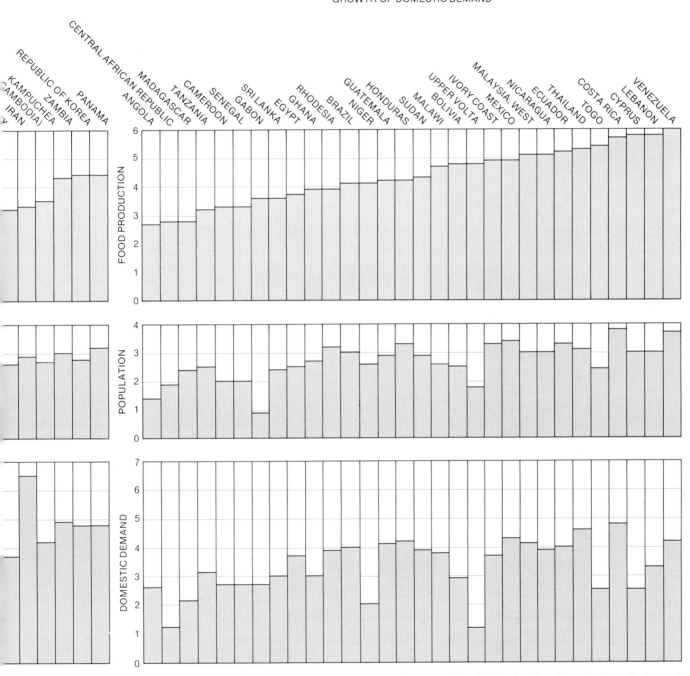

PRODUCTION GROWTH EQUALED OR EXCEEDED
GROWTH OF DOMESTIC DEMAND

through 1971. In the group of 24 nations beginning with Algeria and ending with the Philippines the rise in food production failed to keep pace with the growth of population. In the next 17 nations (Argentina through Panama) the growth of food production exceeded the population growth but fell short of the change in domestic demand. In the final group of 30 nations (from Angola through Venezuela) the rise in food production exceeded population growth and rise in domestic demand. Data are from UN Economic and Social Council.

some catastrophe such as a massive crop failure in the U.S., which is currently the granary of the world.

What of the future? Let us first consider three advances that could be made in dealing with famine. Their common aim is to sight and attack incipient famines in an early stage of development.

The first requirement is an early-warning system. It would employ weather satellites, economic indexes (such as the movement and amounts of food in a region) and clinical indicators. One of the most sensitive clinical indicators is provided by the charted weight and growth curves for children in the most vulnerable socioeconomic sectors of a society.

The second requirement is a permanent small international organization that would keep track of such information for every region and monitor it for any sign of an impending emergency. The agency would maintain manuals on how to proceed against disaster and famine, would hold periodic training sessions for key people from each nation, would draft contingency plans (listing likely requirements and sources of food, medicine, transportation and personnel) and would explore such matters as stockpiling essential supplies and setting up alternative systems of distribution. In an emergency the organization would stand ready to assist a national relief director.

The third requirement is an adequate grain reserve, distributed strategically around the world. It would serve as a standby supply for nearby countries while grain shipments intended for them were diverted to the stricken area. This arrangement might not avert a famine, but it would prevent one from becoming a major disaster.

Several things can also be done to deal with malnutrition. For the next few years it will be necessary to continue to provide food relief where it is needed. The least developed countries may require special assistance in the form of food distribution and feeding programs for some years to come. Those nations should also be helped to develop methods to increase their ability to store food and to distribute it to vulnerable areas in times of emergency.

Simple and inexpensive programs are available to eradicate certain diseases of malnutrition, and they should be instituted. The blindness resulting from a deficiency of vitamin A can be prevented with two injections per year of 100,000 units of the vitamin, at a cost of a few cents per person. Goiter can be prevented by the iodization of salt, also at infinitesimal cost.

In the intermediate term (the next 15 years or so) the goal must be to make the developing nations independent in their food supply. The fish catch appears to have stabilized at the 1970 level. The production of animal foods that compete with human beings for grain should be reduced. (Grazing animals, which utilize land that cannot be cultivated and crops that cannot be eaten by human beings, are another matter.) The development of new foods is still in the future. The only sure resource is the green revolution, which still has the potential of doubling or tripling yields in some areas.

Therefore it is important to begin immediately the construction of fertilizer plants, preferably right at the source of supply (the flare gas around the Persian Gulf and in Nigeria, for example) or in the needy countries. The task should be furthered by international assistance and by oil sold by the OPEC nations at concessional prices.

Another step, which entails something that Americans do well, is to help the food-deficit nations set up agricultural research and extension services, with the aim of adapting the green revolution to a tropical, labor-intensive agriculture and of assisting the small farmer to obtain an increased yield while maintaining a varied production of small animals, fruits and vegetables so that he is not dependent on large tonnages of one crop for an adequate income. Such countries can also be helped to develop ways of protecting a crop once it is har-

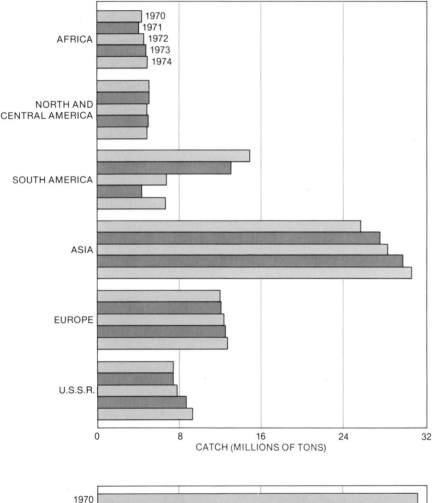

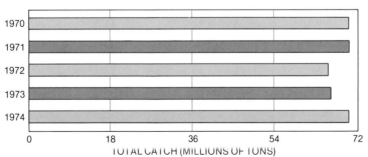

WORLD FISH CATCH appears to have stabilized at about the level of 1970 after declines in 1972 and 1973 that resulted mainly from drops in the South American catch. In most other regions catch has increased slightly. Data are from UN Food and Agriculture Organization.

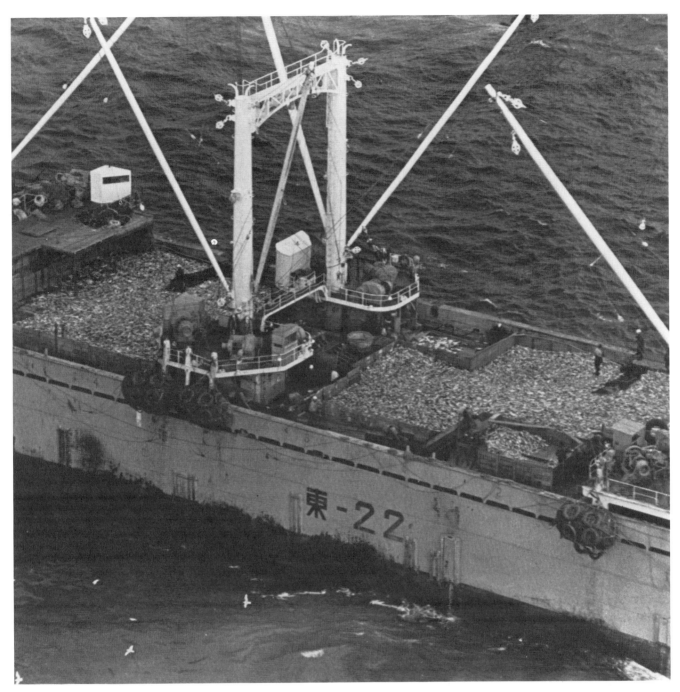

MODERN FISHING METHODS are exemplified by large facto-ry ships such as this Japanese vessel, the *Soyo Maru*. It is a mother **ship for several trawlers, processing their catch while at sea. The fish visible in this photograph of the ship are mainly sole and halibut.**

vested and of establishing an indigenous food industry that can package and distribute the food. A system of international credit that favors the small farmer and the small businessman and promotes a more equitable distribution of income and opportunity should be established. Finally, an international system of weather forecasting should be activated so that future crop failures will not come as a surprise.

These actions will buy time for the next 25 years. If the population of the world is then between six and seven

billion, as seems likely, new sources of food will have to be at hand—on the dinner table, not in the development stage. Unfortunately the nations that will need the new foods the most desperately have neither the financial resources nor the technological skill to do the necessary research, and the nations that do have these things have so far felt no urgency about doing it. The objectives of the research should include the intensive development of aquaculture, the establishment through genetic techniques of new species of animals (such as the beefalo) and of grazing animals

that can utilize forage more efficiently, the domestication of some wild animals, the development of one-cell microorganisms as food and the direct synthesis of food from oil. Work on all these objectives should now be under way.

To sum up, we know who is hungry, if not precisely how many people are affected. We also know why. Economists often say that expanded food production will solve the problem. Social reformers maintain that the need is for more equitable distribution. The evidence shows that we must and can have both.

3

The Requirements of
Human Nutrition

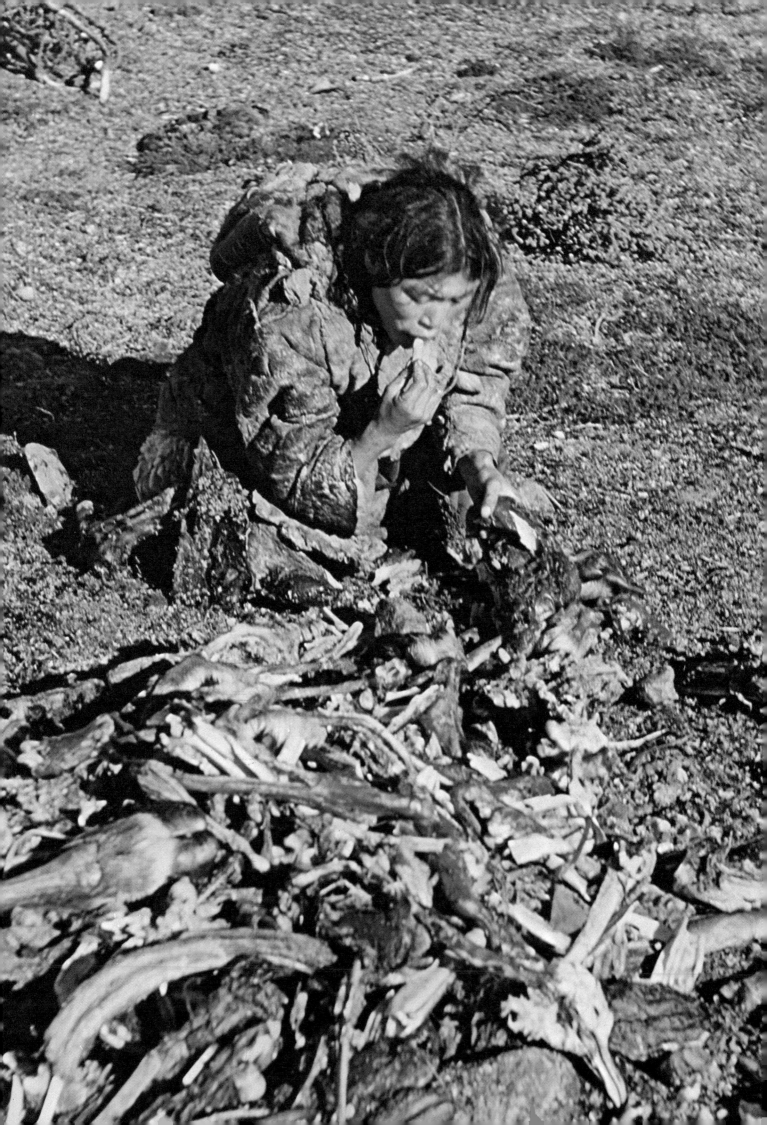

The Requirements of Human Nutrition

NEVIN S. SCRIMSHAW AND VERNON R. YOUNG

Environmental, dietary and physiological factors all interact to set nutritional needs of individuals and populations. Recommended energy and nutrient allowances are thus statistical approximations.

Human beings lack the biochemical machinery to manufacture a variety of carbon compounds required for the formation and maintenance of tissues and for the metabolic reactions that sustain life. These compounds, which all animal cells and organisms must obtain preformed from the environment, together with a number of mineral elements, are termed the essential nutrients. Over the past few million years of evolutionary time the competitive struggle to obtain them in sufficient amounts has favored the emergence and dominance of the human species and has profoundly influenced man's social and cultural ascent. At the same time man's inability to manufacture the essential nutrient compounds has exposed him to deficiency diseases that continue to threaten hundreds of millions of people in today's world.

How did the diverse nutritional requirements of animals, including man, evolve? A significant clue was provided some 30 years ago when the pioneering studies of George W. Beadle and Edward L. Tatum of Stanford University with the red mold *Neurospora* demonstrated that gene mutation can bring about alterations in the needs of cells and organisms for an external supply of compounds. Like all other plants, *Neurospora* normally requires no vitamins or amino acids for its metabolism and growth; it makes them itself. When Beadle and Tatum exposed the mold cells to X rays, however, the resulting mutations caused a loss in the cells' ability to synthesize vitamins such as thiamine, pyridoxine and para-aminobenzoic acid and the amino acids histidine, lysine and tryptophan.

Evolutionary biologists now believe a similar series of mutations occurred in the remote past to give rise to the nutrient-synthesizing deficiencies of animals. The earliest forms of life appear to have been simple bacteriumlike organisms that were capable of manufacturing all the compounds they needed from mineral salts, nitrogen, simple compounds of carbon and of course water. This ability entailed the storage of an enormous amount of genetic information, and cells that could reduce the metabolic costs of replicating and maintaining genes gained a selective advantage. With natural selection favoring mutations that eliminated the "unnecessary" enzymatic synthesis of readily available nutrients, primitive forms of life evolved and ultimately developed into animal cells.

When the first single-cell animals appeared about a billion years ago, they lacked a number of the biosynthetic pathways found in plant cells, notably the photosynthetic pathway that enables a plant to convert the energy of sunlight into the energy-rich compounds that drive the metabolism of cells. All the animal species that subsequently emerged from these ancestral beginnings had similar deficiencies, but they survived by obtaining the energy and nutrients they needed from external sources. For example, plants have retained the ability to make all the 20 amino acids found in their proteins from simple carbon and nitrogen compounds, whereas animals depend on their diet to supply about half of these amino acids.

An interesting and quite recent evolutionary development of nutritional significance is the inability of certain animals to synthesize ascorbic acid (vitamin C). I. B. Chatterjee of the University College of Science in India has estimated that some 350 million years ago the capacity for synthesizing this vitamin arose in amphibians, but that a gene mutation about 25 million years ago in a common ancestor of man and other primates led to a loss of the enzyme L-gulono oxidase, which catalyzed the terminal step in the conversion of glucose to ascorbic acid. Linus Pauling has suggested that the loss of this pathway was selectively advantageous in that it freed glucose for energy use by the body. In any case the mutation was not lethal because the missing compound was present in the food of the mutant animals. Their evolution could thus continue.

Man's need to obtain an adequate supply of essential nutrients through his diet not only is a part of his biological evolution but also has shaped his social evolution. It has been suggested that the migration of human groups to the northern regions of the earth was slowed by the limited amounts of ascorbic acid in the foods available in those areas during the long winter months. Moreover, man's dependence on an adequate supply of nutrients meant that he initially had to be a hunter and gatherer, which circumscribed his cultural development. With the domestication of the cereal grains and other plants, along with a limited number of animal species, he was able to organize a stable way of life and secure the essential nutrients without foraging over substantial areas. This freed his energies for new kinds of so-

PREGNANT CARIBOU ESKIMO WOMAN chews caribou bones to extract the last scraps of nutrient-rich marrow in this photograph made in 1955 by Fritz Goro in the Canadian Northwest Territories. Scattered over barren taiga south of the Arctic Circle, small bands of these inland Eskimos subsisted entirely on the caribou, relying on the animal for food and clothing and even using the bones for projectile points and other tools. Although the caribou were once plentiful, in the late 1950's they changed their migration route, causing a disastrous famine among the Caribou Eskimos. In 1960 the Canadian government airlifted the survivors to the coast, where they mixed with other Eskimos and went to work in a nickel mine. Today the Caribou Eskimos do not exist as a distinct population, victims of their single-source diet.

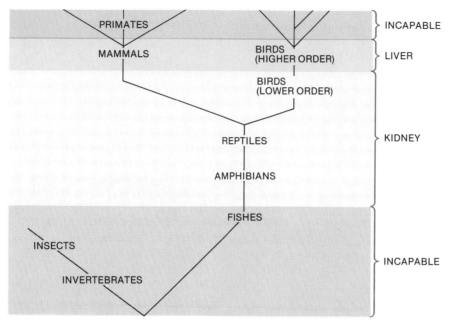

ABILITY OF ANIMALS TO SYNTHESIZE VITAMIN C and the type of cell performing the synthesis have varied over the span of evolution. Some 25 million years ago a mutation in an ancestor of primates (including man) and other mammals resulted in a loss of the terminal enzyme in the synthetic pathway. For this reason primates, guinea pigs, bats and some birds require a dietary source of the vitamin to prevent development of nutritional disease.

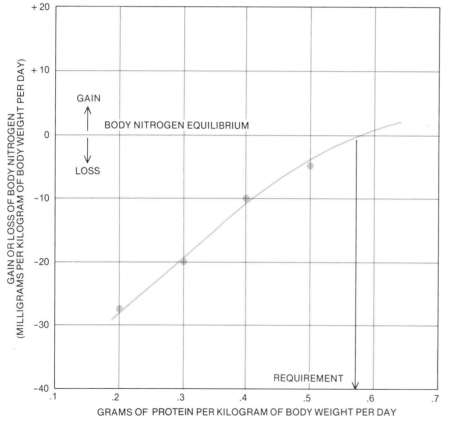

MINIMUM PROTEIN REQUIREMENT for a population of privileged young men was determined in the authors' laboratory with the metabolic-balance technique. Students at the Massachusetts Institute of Technology were studied at various protein (nitrogen) intakes for 15-day periods. They received a constant diet in which the entire protein source was whole dried-egg powder. Nitrogen-balance values (intake minus excretion equals balance) for the seven subjects were measured at each intake level; data points shown are statistical mean of individual numbers. Amount of protein sufficient to maintain nitrogen balance, where subjects were neither losing nor gaining body nitrogen, was judged to be minimum requirement.

cial, economic and artistic activities.

At least 45 and possibly as many as 50 dietary compounds and elements are now recognized as essential for a human being to live a full, healthy life. Plant and animal foods cannot, however, be directly utilized by the cells of human tissues. The nutrients contained in foods are released by digestion, absorbed in the intestine and transported to the cells by the blood. As long as the overall diet supplies all the essential nutrients, the cells and tissues of the body are capable of synthesizing the many thousands of additional compounds required for life.

Since the body is dependent on a regular supply of nutrients, intricate biochemical mechanisms have evolved to regulate the availability of the nutrients to the cells so that the organism can adjust to a wide range of intakes. Those nutrients that have been acquired in excess of cellular needs are handled by catabolic pathways that bring about their breakdown. The breakdown products are then eliminated in the urine, bile, sweat and other body secretions so that they do not accumulate and reach toxic levels.

The importance of regulating nutrient levels is dramatically illustrated in certain human diseases. In the genetic disorder known as maple-syrup-urine disease infants cannot adequately metabolize the branched-chain amino acids (leucine, isoleucine and valine). In another genetic disorder, phenylketonuria, the enzyme for breaking down the amino acid phenylalanine is lacking. Both conditions cause a buildup of amino acids in the blood and the tissues, particularly the brain, leading to cell death and mental retardation. The management of patients with these diseases consists of special diets containing a low level of the offending nutrient.

Another example of the accumulation of nutrients to toxic levels is hemochromatosis, a severe form of liver disease usually resulting from a combination of high iron and alcohol intakes that give rise to an excessive accumulation of iron in the liver. Vitamins A, D and K are also toxic in high concentrations. Hypervitaminosis from an excessive dietary intake of vitamin A, usually from the misguided use of high-potency vitamin pills, results in thickening of the skin, headaches and increased susceptibility to disease.

On the other hand, if the nutrient intake is so low that it is insufficient to meet the normal needs of cells, changes occur within the cells and tissues that act to conserve the limited supply. These changes may involve a more effective absorption of nutrients from the intestine and the activation of biochemical mechanisms that enhance the retention of the nutrient once it is inside the body.

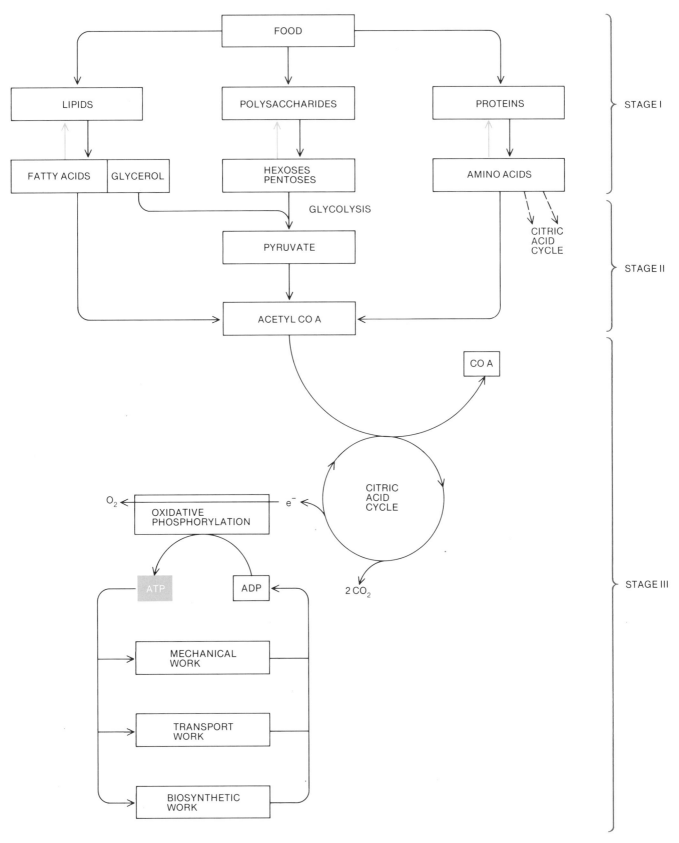

METABOLISM OF ENERGY-CONTAINING NUTRIENTS in the body proceeds in three major stages. In the first stage the large nutrient molecules of food are degraded into their main building blocks by digestive enzymes in the alimentary tract. In the second stage the many different products of the first stage are absorbed by the intestine and transported by the blood to the tissue cells. There they can either be incorporated into cellular molecules by anabolic pathways (*colored arrows*) or converted by catabolic pathways into a small number of intermediates that play a central role in metabolism. Glucose, glycerol, fatty acids and many amino acids are converted into a single two-carbon species: the acetyl group of the carrier molecule coenzyme A (CoA). In the third stage, which is localized in the mitochondria of cells, coenzyme A brings acetyl units into the citric acid cycle, where they are completely oxidized to carbon dioxide, concurrently releasing four pairs of electrons. The energy-rich compound adenosine triphosphate (ATP) is generated as the electrons flow down a transport chain to oxygen, the ultimate electron acceptor. Oxidation of a single glucose molecule can result in the formation of 36 molecules of ATP. Once generated, ATP provides the energy for the numerous physiological and synthetic activities of cells.

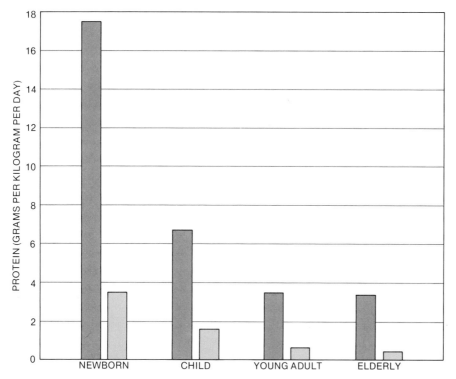

DECLINE IN DIETARY PROTEIN REQUIREMENT per unit of body weight (*color*) approximately parallels the change in rate of whole-body protein synthesis during the stages of life (*gray*). The early phase of rapid development in infants requires high levels of protein turnover and dietary intake, but both fall off as the rate of growth decreases. (Since 70 percent or more of the amino acids utilized in protein synthesis are provided by breakdown of other body proteins, dietary need is small in relation to turnover.) Data for infants, young adults and elderly subjects were obtained at the Clinical Research Center at M.I.T.; those for one-year-old children were provided by D. Picou of the Tropical Metabolism Research Unit in Jamaica.

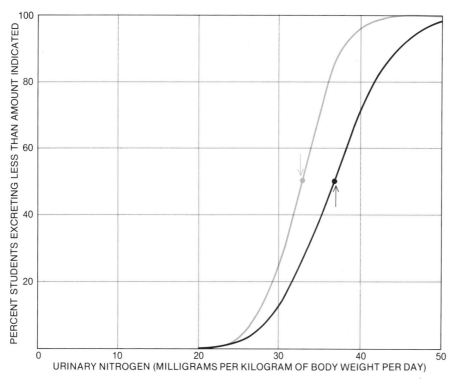

VARIATION IN PROTEIN METABOLISM of two genetically and geographically different population groups was revealed to a statistically significant degree by the distribution of obligatory urinary nitrogen losses in young men fed on a protein-free diet for 12 days. Daily urinary nitrogen excretion during the last four days of the experimental period was measured in 83 male college students studied at M.I.T. by the authors (*black curve*) and in 50 students subsequently studied by P.-C. Huang at the National Taiwan University College of Medicine (*colored curve*). The graph shows the mean excretion for each population (*vertical arrows*) and the cumulative distribution of urinary nitrogen losses within the two groups of students.

If the dietary intake continues to be inadequate, these metabolic adaptations break down and deficiency disease rises above the "clinical horizon," with characteristic symptoms that can lead to disability and death.

In addition to essential nutrients the body needs a supply of energy, that is, energy-rich compounds whose energy content is measured in calories. The assessment of the quantitative requirements for calories and the essential nutrients is clearly of great practical importance in human nutrition. The task is far more difficult than is generally realized. In animal husbandry the minimum needs of the animal for individual nutrients can be judged in relation to certain productive functions, such as rapid growth in meat-producing animals, high milk yield in dairy cows and maximum fleece production in sheep. The nutrient requirements of the human organism cannot be defined as readily because its well-being is more difficult to measure. What are the appropriate yardsticks? Maximum physical fitness and disease resistance would seem to be logical criteria for assessing the requirements for individual nutrients, but because we cannot quantify physical well-being as precisely as we can the growth of experimental animals, we must seek more objective measures.

Some nutrients or their breakdown products are excreted daily in the urine, feces and sweat and are lost through the shedding of small amounts of skin and hair. For the body to remain in metabolic equilibrium the total gain of a nutrient in food must equal the total loss. Therefore by measuring the intake required to balance the amount lost daily by the body it is possible to estimate the minimum metabolic need for a given nutrient. For example, nitrogen, a characteristic and relatively constant component of protein, is measured to determine protein needs. The metabolic-balance approach has also been followed in measuring the requirements for calcium, zinc and magnesium, but it is not suited to nutrients that are oxidized and whose carbon is eliminated in the respired air, such as fats and vitamins. For those nutrients the requirement can be estimated by determining the minimum amount of the nutrient that prevents the onset of subclinical deficiency disease, although the technique has its methodological and ethical restrictions.

Even when the metabolic-balance method is applicable, it does not provide information on where in the body the nutrient is being retained or utilized; overall nutrient balance might be achieved with a given intake of the nutrient being examined, but this does not prove that the tissues are functioning optimally and that health will be maintained. In addition it is difficult to carry out balance studies for prolonged dietary periods; such studies call for sophisticated facilities and a team of trained workers. The need to carefully control nutrient-intake levels requires that the daily menu be monotonous. Losses in the urine and feces (and ideally in sweat, skin and hair as well) must be assayed quantitatively, which means additional inconvenience for the subjects and technical problems for the investigators, particularly when the subjects are infants, young children or elderly people. For these reasons metabolic-balance studies are usually of short duration: a week or less in children and two or three weeks in adults. The long-term nutritional and health significance of these brief study periods has not been critically determined, so that the adequacy of our current estimates of nutrient requirements, which have been based on short-term studies, is uncertain. This is not a satisfactory state of affairs.

In the Department of Nutrition and Food Science at the Massachusetts Institute of Technology, working with Edwina E. Murray as research nutritionist and several physician graduate students, we have been able to complete a series of long-term metabolic-balance studies with highly motivated and cooperative students. These subjects have adhered to monotonous diets and have followed strict regimens for the complete daily collection of urine and feces for periods lasting up to 100 days, a significant increase over the usual 14- to 21-day balance period.

In one study six volunteer subjects lived on a diet providing protein at a level equal to the safe practical intake recommended by the 1973 Joint Food and Agriculture Organization–World Health Organization Expert Committee on Energy and Protein Requirements. By the end of three months metabolic measurements on these subjects indicated that there were decreases in lean body and muscle mass and/or changes in liver metabolism. These results

IRON IS RELEASED FROM FOODS during digestion. In the ferrous (Fe^{++}) oxidation state it passes from within the intestine into the cells of the intestinal mucosa, where it is oxidized to the ferric (Fe^{+++}) form. Ferric ion then combines with the protein apoferritin to form the complex known as ferritin. The amount of iron bound up in ferritin at any given time helps to stabilize the level of iron in the blood and protect the cells from iron toxicity. At the surface of the mucosal cell ferric ion is reduced to the ferrous form and enters the bloodstream, where it is reoxidized. It then combines with the protein transferrin, which transports it to the various tissues. Relatively little iron is excreted; the iron liberated by the breakdown of hemoglobin is recycled for the manufacture of hemoglobin.

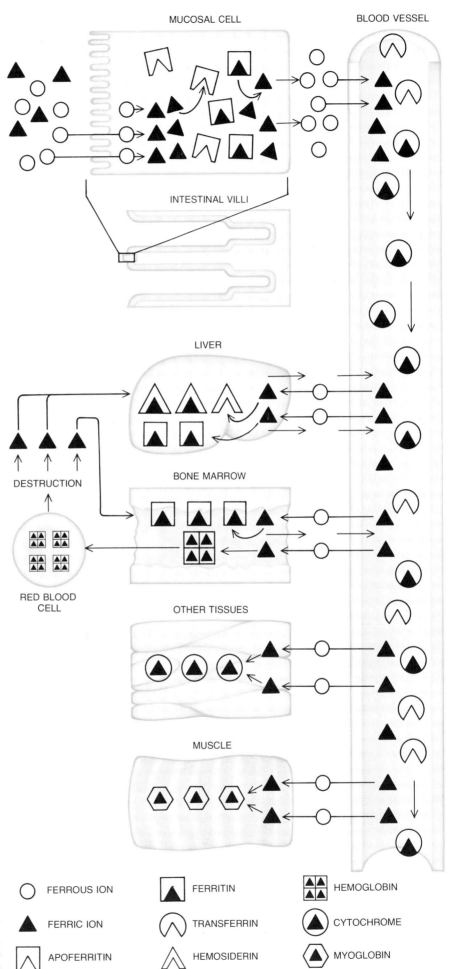

MUCOSAL CELL
BLOOD VESSEL
INTESTINAL VILLI
LIVER
DESTRUCTION
BONE MARROW
RED BLOOD CELL
OTHER TISSUES
MUSCLE

⃝ FERROUS ION ◻◣ FERRITIN ▦ HEMOGLOBIN
▲ FERRIC ION ⌓ TRANSFERRIN CYTOCHROME
⌂ APOFERRITIN △ HEMOSIDERIN ⬡ MYOGLOBIN

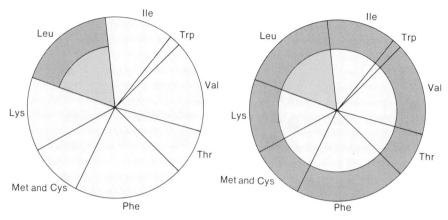

NINE ESSENTIAL AMINO ACIDS must be present simultaneously and in correct relative amounts for protein synthesis to occur. If one or more of the essential amino acids are partially missing (*dark color*), the utilization of all other amino acids in the cellular pool will be reduced in the same proportion. Leftover amino acids cannot be stored and are metabolized for energy. The amino acid abbreviations are Leu, leucine; Val, valine; Phe, phenylalanine; Thr, threonine; Ile, isoleucine; Lys, lysine; Met, methionine; Cys, cystine; Trp, tryptophan.

strongly suggest that short-term metabolic balance studies are not sufficient as the sole criterion for assessing human protein requirements and that the current recommendations for dietary protein intake for large population groups are inadequate. Although our own balance studies have involved experimental diet periods significantly longer than those employed for the FAO–WHO estimates, the fact remains that the experimental subjects are few in number and are confined to privileged American males, and that the duration of the study is still limited.

For some of the essential nutrients none of these approaches has been followed, and only vague epidemiological data are available. Here we must depend mainly on data obtained in animal

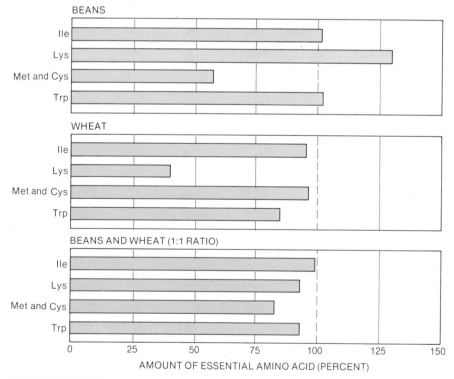

PROTEIN COMPLEMENTARITY can come about when a "poor quality" protein inadequate in certain essential amino acids but adequate in others is mixed with another protein having opposite strengths and weaknesses. If the two kinds of protein are ingested simultaneously or within a short time, the mixture can yield an overall amino acid balance comparable to that of a "high quality" protein ingested alone. The broken line represents 100 percent of the essential amino acid levels in a standard reference protein that is considered by a Food and Agriculture Organization–World Health Organization expert committee to best meet human requirements. Complementary protein combinations are found in almost all cultures.

experiments and extrapolate the results cautiously to humans, or attempt to assess how much well-nourished groups consume and consider that as an adequate intake level.

The many difficulties faced in determining the amounts of nutrients required by an individual are compounded by the problem of determining the variation in the requirements of that individual over a period of time, and with the variation encountered among individuals. It is easy to establish that physiological states such as growth, pregnancy and lactation call for greater amounts of most nutrients than those needed by healthy adults for maintenance alone. It is harder to measure the subtle changes in requirements that occur in the aging adult, a problem often complicated by the cumulative effects of both acute and chronic diseases that can affect requirements for nutrients by interfering with their absorption or utilization.

Knowledge of nutrient requirements in infants and in young children is also on uncertain ground. There is a tendency for investigators to regard such individuals as little adults and, with a small allowance for their growth, to extrapolate their requirements proportionally by weight from studies of older individuals. This approach does not take into account changes in the metabolic activities of cells and in the rates of nutrient turnover with age. For body protein, studies in our laboratory demonstrate high rates of turnover in newborn infants that diminish rapidly during the early weeks and months of infancy. Thereafter the decline is less rapid, but on a whole-body basis it probably continues with the passage of time during the adult years. Although protein requirements are not determined entirely by metabolic-turnover rate, the direction of change in the requirements for total dietary protein is the same as that for body protein turnover.

There is also variation in nutrient requirements among individuals of the same age, sex and physiological state because of the interaction of genetic and environmental factors. The important variation in nutritional requirements is the one that is due to the actual expression of genes in the individual, rather than the potential expression of genes under ideal circumstances. For example, in Japan there has been an increase in the height of adults over the past 30 years, when a progressively greater proportion of the full genetic potential was expressed as dietary and environmental conditions improved.

One problem in knowing the appropriate variation to assign to nutrient requirements in normal individuals is the lack of data on the populations of different countries. In a study at M.I.T. we have given students a protein-free but otherwise adequate diet for 12 days in order to estimate the minimum level of nitrogen excretion, known as the obligatory loss. The statistical means of this urinary nitrogen value were significantly higher than those found subsequently for university students in Taiwan, who were studied under comparable conditions by P.-C. Huang of the National Taiwan University College of Medicine. Whether this disparity is due to genetic differences or to environmental and experimental factors is currently undetermined, but the fact of the difference appears to be indisputable. The nutritional significance of this observation is not fully known, but it emphasizes the great need for a larger number of comparative studies on nutrient metabolism and requirements in populations of differing geographic, cultural and genetic backgrounds.

Nutrient requirements also depend on a variety of environmental factors that may be physical (for example average ambient temperature), biological (the presence of infectious organisms and other parasites) or social (physical activity, the type of clothing worn, sanitary conditions and personal hygiene and other patterns of behavior). Environmental factors can influence nutritional status by directly modifying dietary requirements or by their effects on the production and availability of food and on its consumption.

The major dietary factors influencing nutrient requirements are threefold. The first is that the form of a nutrient in food may have a significant effect on its degree of absorption and utilization. For example, the relatively low efficiency of the absorption of iron from vegetable foods is a major factor in the total iron intake required by human beings. Ferrous iron (reduced iron, as in ferrous sulfate or finely divided elemental iron) is more effectively absorbed than ferric iron (as in ferric chloride or iron pyrophosphate). Even ferrous iron, however, is absorbed less efficiently when it is ingested in combination with phytates and oxalates, which are found in leafy green vegetables and the whole-grain, unleav-

NET PROTEIN UTILIZATION values are an index of the "quality," or nutritional value, of proteins from various food sources. They are the percent of the amino acids ingested as protein that are retained in the body and incorporated into cellular proteins. Egg protein, along with that of milk and most meats, has excellent proportions of all the essential amino acids, and its net utilization by the body is accordingly high. Legumes, on the other hand, are deficient in one or more of the nine essential amino acids, which greatly reduces the proportion of total amino acids that are available for protein synthesis and thus gives rise to their low NPU values.

FOOD	ESSENTIAL AMINO ACIDS		NET PROTEIN UTILIZATION (PERCENT) 0 25 50 75 100
	POOR	ADEQUATE	
DAIRY			
EGGS	—	Trp, Lys, Met, Cys	
COW'S MILK	—	Trp, Lys	
COTTAGE CHEESE	—	Lys	
SWISS CHEESE	—	Lys	
MEATS			
FISH	—	Lys	
TURKEY	—	Lys	
PORK	—	Lys	
BEEF	—	Lys	
CHICKEN	—	Lys	
LAMB	—	Lys	
VEGETABLES			
CORN	Trp, Lys	—	
ASPARAGUS	Met, Cys	—	
BROCCOLI	Met, Cys	—	
CAULIFLOWER	Met, Cys	Trp, Lys	
POTATO	Met, Cys	Trp	
KALE	Lys, Met, Cys	—	
GREEN PEAS	Met, Cys	Lys	
GRAINS AND CEREALS			
BROWN RICE	Lys	—	
WHEAT GERM	Trp	Lys	
OATMEAL	Lys	—	
WHEAT GRAIN	Lys	—	
RYE	Trp, Lys	—	
POLISHED RICE	Lys, Thr	Trp	
MILLET	Lys	Trp, Met, Cys	
PASTA	Lys, Met, Cys	—	
LEGUMES			
SOYBEANS	Met, Cys, Val	Lys, Trp	
LIMA BEANS	Met, Cys	Trp, Lys	
KIDNEY BEANS	Trp, Met, Cys	Lys	
LENTILS	Trp, Met, Cys	Lys	
NUTS AND SEEDS			
SUNFLOWER SEEDS	Lys	Trp	
SESAME SEEDS	Lys	Trp, Met, Cys	
PEANUTS	Lys, Met, Cys, Thr	—	

34

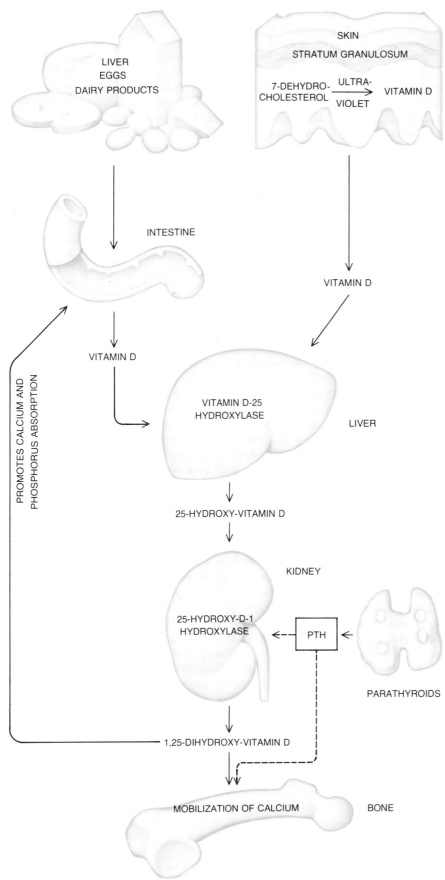

LIVER
EGGS
DAIRY PRODUCTS

SKIN

STRATUM GRANULOSUM

7-DEHYDRO-CHOLESTEROL → ULTRA-VIOLET → VITAMIN D

INTESTINE

VITAMIN D

VITAMIN D

PROMOTES CALCIUM AND PHOSPHORUS ABSORPTION

VITAMIN D

VITAMIN D-25 HYDROXYLASE

LIVER

25-HYDROXY-VITAMIN D

KIDNEY

25-HYDROXY-D-1 HYDROXYLASE ← PTH ←

PARATHYROIDS

1,25-DIHYDROXY-VITAMIN D

MOBILIZATION OF CALCIUM

BONE

VITAMIN D is absorbed preformed from certain foods and is also synthesized in the stratum granulosum of the skin through the action of solar radiation on the closely related steroid 7-dehydrocholesterol. The physiological roles of the vitamin depend on its conversion to the active form 1,25-dihydroxy-vitamin D, which occurs in two enzyme-catalyzed steps, the first in the liver and the second in the kidney. Parathyroid hormone (PTH) serves to regulate the synthesis of the active form of the vitamin, and both act to mobilize calcium from bone. In addition the dihydroxylated vitamin alone stimulates calcium absorption from the small intestine.

ened bread of North Africa and the Middle East. The iron found in meat (heme iron) is much better absorbed than iron of vegetable origin, and small amounts of red meat markedly improve overall iron absorption.

The second major factor affecting nutrient requirements is that the presence or absence of one nutrient frequently affects the utilization of another. For example, when dietary protein intake is deficient, the two proteins that play a role in the transport of vitamin A (retinol-binding protein and prealbumin) are not made by the liver in adequate amounts. The esterified form of the vitamin remains stored in the liver, unavailable to the other body tissues. Signs of vitamin-A deficiency may then appear, in spite of the fact that the intake of the vitamin (or of its precursor, beta-carotene, which is present in plant foods) would be sufficient if protein nutrition were adequate.

The third factor is the presence in the human large intestine of bacteria that live on organic molecules not absorbed in the small intestine. In the course of their metabolic activities these bacteria manufacture vitamins that their human host absorbs; it is a symbiotic, or mutually beneficial, relationship. Vitamin K, a deficiency of which causes failure of blood clotting, is synthesized in this way, as are small quantities of some of the B vitamins.

The factors influencing the adequacy of dietary protein for an individual may be even more complex. In the first place, the normal requirement is not for protein per se but, depending on the individual's age, for some nine or 10 essential amino acids in adequate amounts and appropriate proportions. Whether an amino acid is utilized for the synthesis of new protein or is degraded for its energy content (a wasteful process) depends on a number of factors. First, each of the essential amino acids must be present simultaneously in the intracellular pool for protein synthesis to proceed. If a given amino acid is present only in a limited amount, the protein can be formed only as long as the supply of that amino acid (called the limiting amino acid) lasts. If one essential amino acid is missing from the pool, the remaining ones cannot be stored for later synthesis and will be catabolized for energy.

The level of nonprotein calories in the diet is also important. If it is high with respect to need, the ingested protein is spared from breakdown to meet energy requirements, but the individual tends to become obese. If it is low, some of the protein will be preempted to meet energy requirements and will not be available to fulfill the actual protein needs of the body. It is sometimes mistakenly believed that it is not worth improving the protein content of a diet if caloric intake is deficient. Our studies of young adults indicate that some improvement in protein retention is achieved even under circumstances of deficient energy intake. Adequate nonspecific sources of nitrogen are also needed so that the nonessential amino acids and other metabolically important nitrogenous compounds can be synthesized in the body.

Various proteins differ in their essential amino acid concentration and balance. A nutritionally "complete" protein source such as meat, eggs or milk supplies enough of all the essential amino acids needed to meet the body's requirements for maintenance and growth. A low-quality or nutritionally "incomplete" protein such as the zein of corn, which lacks the amino acids tryptophan and lysine, cannot support either maintenance or growth. A somewhat less inferior protein such as the gliadin of wheat provides enough lysine for maintenance but not enough for growth. Plant proteins usually contain inadequate amounts of one essential amino acid or more. Lysine and threonine levels in cereals are generally low, and corn is also deficient in tryptophan. Legumes are good sources of lysine but are low in the sulfur-containing amino acids methionine and cystine; leafy green vegetables are well balanced in all the essential amino acids except methionine.

In spite of these shortcomings of individual foods it is possible to devise meals containing acceptable proportions of essential amino acids by combining proteins from several sources. In general, cereals that are deficient in lysine are complemented by legumes that are deficient in methionine. Every culture has evolved its own mixtures of complementary proteins. In the Middle East wheat bread, which lacks adequate levels of lysine, is eaten with cheese, which has a high lysine content. Mexicans eat beans and rice, Jamaicans eat rice and peas, Indians eat wheat and pulses, and Americans eat breakfast cereals with milk. This kind of supplementation, particularly in infants and growing children, only works, however, when the deficient and complementary proteins are ingested together or are ingested separately within a few hours.

Acute or chronic infections or other disease processes that cause decreased gastrointestinal function increase the need for dietary protein, because less of it will be absorbed. Trauma, anxiety, fear and other causes of stress have an even more pronounced effect in altering protein requirements. Stress results in an increase in the catabolism of muscle protein with respect to synthesis, leading to the transport of amino acids away from muscle and peripheral tissues to the liver, where they are converted to glucose for energy pur-

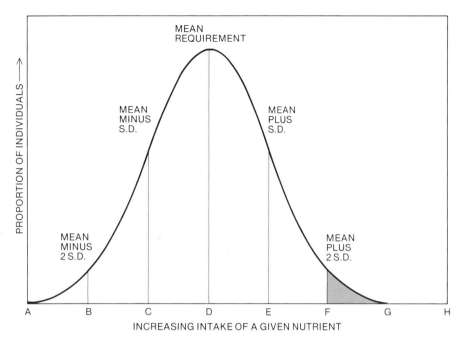

DISTRIBUTION OF NUTRIENT REQUIREMENTS in a hypothetical population of healthy individuals is bell-shaped. *D* is the mean requirement for the population. The statistical unit of variation from the mean is known as the standard deviation (S.D.), which is calculated from the sum of the squares of each individual's replacement values, minus the square of the average value, divided by the square root of the total number of observations. An intake of *F*, obtained by adding two standard deviations to the mean value, would cover the requirements for nearly all (97.5 percent) of the individuals in this population. Colored region shows the small minority of healthy individuals (2.5 percent) not covered by the allowance. This approach has been followed by international committees in estimating dietary allowances.

poses. This process creates a deficit in the protein content of the body, which must be compensated for by increased protein retention during the recovery period.

With any infection, even immunization with live-virus vaccines, there is a loss of appetite that leads to a decrease in food intake. The metabolic consequences of acute infections have been most extensively documented by William R. Beisel and his collaborators at the Army Medical Research Institute of Infectious Diseases. The first changes are increased synthesis of antibodies and other proteins characteristic of acute illness, followed by catabolic responses that result in increased losses of nitrogen (from body protein), vitamin A, vitamin C, iron and zinc, and probably other nutrients as well.

Disease may also directly upset the mechanisms controlling the metabolism of essential nutrients, thereby altering dietary nutrient requirements. The conversion of vitamin D into its metabolically active form, for example, depends on the activities of the liver and the kidneys. If the kidneys are diseased, the normal utilization of the vitamin is compromised. It is for this reason that many individuals suffering from kidney disease show skeletal abnormalities similar to those seen in rickets, a disease of vitamin D deficiency. When these patients are given a synthetic form of the active

derivative of the vitamin, they show a marked improvement in health.

The absorption of nutrients is reduced whenever the gastrointestinal tract is significantly affected by acute or chronic infections, by a high concentration of intestinal parasites or by malaria (which interferes with the mesenteric circulation). Chronic infections and parasitic infestations are also capable of increasing nutrient requirements in other ways. Even with a diet that would otherwise be adequate iron-deficiency anemia can develop as a result of the intestinal blood loss associated with hookworm, schistosomiasis and certain protozoal infections. In northern European countries where the eating of raw fish commonly leads to heavy infestations of fish tapeworm, vitamin B-12 deficiency disease (anemia and neurological damage) often develops in affected individuals because the parasite has a particularly large requirement for the vitamin.

For these reasons young children in developing countries who are subject to intestinal, respiratory and other infections that increase nutrient requirements, and who at the same time have a poor diet, are particularly likely to develop acute nutritional disease. The ideal public-health approach would be to eliminate the infections rather than to provide the extra amounts of nutrients these conditions require, but that is frequently not possible because of a lack of resources or for social reasons. All these sources of variation in nutrient requirements make it impossible to generate precise values for nutrient requirements in either individuals or population groups. Instead nutrient allowances must be viewed statistically, on the assumption that individual variation in a nutrient requirement is distributed in a bell-shaped curve above and below the mean requirement for that population group.

It is not practical to attempt to arrive at nutritional recommendations sufficient to cover 100 percent of a population, because this would require far more nutrition than is necessary for most people. There will always be a few normal individuals in a population, two or three per 100, who need more of a nutrient than can be recommended in

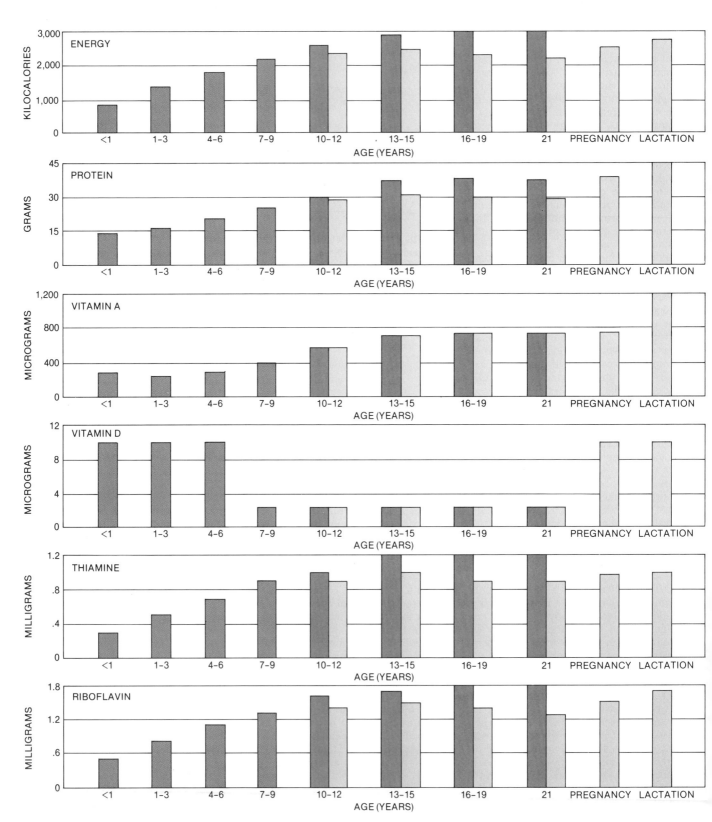

RECOMMENDED DAILY ALLOWANCES for energy, protein and selected vitamins and minerals shown here were agreed on by an FAO–WHO expert committee in 1974. Requirements vary markedly with age, and those of males (*gray*) are significantly different from

a practical dietary allowance, and a smaller number at the extreme tail of the bell curve, two or three per 1,000, whose metabolic abnormalities significantly increase their requirements. Finally, recommended daily allowances (RDA's) are intended only to cover healthy individuals and are often not adequate for people suffering from acute or chronic diseases.

The major limitation to the practical use of RDA's is that they are based on data from small and possibly unrepresentative samples that have been extrap- olated to populations of all types. In developing countries, where a large fraction of the population is likely to be suffering from disease, children have a greatly reduced weight and height for their age because of the combined effects of repeated infections and malnu-

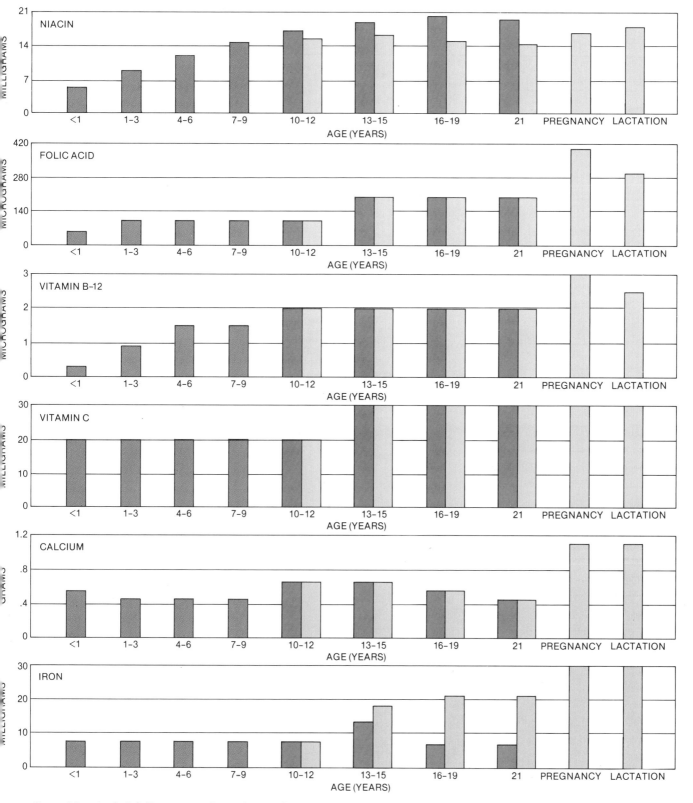

those of females (*color*). Pregnancy and lactation also increase nutritional needs. Recommended allowances are not absolute for individuals; they can be justifiably applied only to reasonably healthy populations and may well be subject to revision as knowledge advances.

trition. As a result the body size of adults is also small. For them the age-specific nutritional figures derived from well-nourished populations may be unnecessarily high and estimated caloric requirements may be excessive. It is therefore preferable to calculate allowances for adults in developing countries on the basis of kilograms of body weight.

Per-kilogram allowances are not sufficient, however, for children whose growth has been stunted by malnutrition and disease. Such allowances will be too low for maximum catch-up growth and will perpetuate the existing poor nutritional state of the children. A compromise in countries where nutritional dwarfism among children is common is to estimate the specific requirements of children on a per kilogram

ESSENTIAL AMINO ACIDS	RDA FOR HEALTHY ADULT MALE (MILLIGRAMS)	DIETARY SOURCES	MAJOR BODY FUNCTIONS	DEFICIENCY	EXCESS
AROMATIC					
PHENYLALANINE	1,100				
TYROSINE					
BASIC					
LYSINE	800				
HISTIDINE	Not known				

BRANCHED CHAIN		FROM PROTEINS
		
		GOOD SOURCES
		  Legume grains
		  Dairy products
		  Meat
		  Fish
			Precursors of structural protein, enzymes, antibodies, hormones, metabolically active compounds
			
			Certain amino acids have specific functions:
				Deficient protein intake leads to development of kwashiorkor and, coupled with low energy intake, to marasmus.	Excess protein intake possibly aggravates or potentiates chronic disease states.

ISOLEUCINE	700		(a) Tyrosine is a precursor of epinephrine and thyroxine		

LEUCINE	1,000	ADEQUATE SOURCES
		  Rice
		  Corn
		  Wheat
			(b) Arginine is a precursor of polyamines		

VALINE	800	POOR SOURCES
		  Cassava
		  Sweet potato
			(c) Methionine is required for methyl group metabolism
			(d) Tryptophan is a precursor of serotonin		

SULFUR-CONTAINING					
METHIONINE	1,100				
CYSTINE					
OTHER					
TRYPTOPHAN	250				
THREONINE	500				
ESSENTIAL FATTY ACIDS					
ARACHIDONIC		Vegetable fats (corn, cottonseed, soy oils) Wheat germ Vegetable shortenings	Involved in cell membrane structure and function. Precursors of prostaglandins (regulation of gastric function, release of hormones, smooth-muscle activity)	Poor growth Skin lesions	Not known
LINOLEIC	6,000				
LINOLENIC					

ESSENTIAL AMINO ACIDS AND FATTY ACIDS cannot be synthesized in the body and must be present in food. Amino acids are the building blocks of body proteins; essential fatty acids are involved in the maintenance of cell membrane structure and function and serve as precursors of the prostaglandins, a family of hormone-like compounds that have diverse physiological actions in the body.

basis and add a modest extra allowance for catch-up growth.

When acute infections are prevalent in a population, extra allowance must be made for the individual during recovery, although because of reduced food intake during the acute phase of the illness and increased retention of some nutrients in depleted individuals, the overall food requirements of the group suffering from infections may be little affected. Increased dietary allowances may nonetheless be needed to compensate for continuing high nutrient losses or for the impaired absorption associated with intestinal-parasite load and chronic disease.

In sum, recommended allowances cannot serve as an absolute indicator of the adequacy of a given intake for a given individual. They can justifiably be

VITAMIN	RDA FOR HEALTHY ADULT MALE (MILLIGRAMS)	DIETARY SOURCES	MAJOR BODY FUNCTIONS	DEFICIENCY	EXCESS
WATER-SOLUBLE					
VITAMIN B-1 (THIAMINE)	1.5	Pork, organ meats, whole grains, legumes	Coenzyme (thiamine pyrophosphate) in reactions involving the removal of carbon dioxide.	Beriberi (peripheral nerve changes, edema, heart failure)	None reported
VITAMIN B-2 (RIBOFLAVIN)	1.8	Widely distributed in foods.	Constituent of two flavin nucleotide coenzymes involved in energy metabolism (FAD and FMN)	Reddened lips, cracks at corner of mouth (cheilosis), lesions of eye	None reported
NIACIN	20	Liver, lean meats, grains, legumes (can be formed from tryptophan)	Constituent of two coenzymes involved in oxidation-reduction reactions (NAD and NADP)	Pellagra (skin and gastrointestinal lesions, nervous, mental disorders)	Flushing, burning and tingling around neck, face and hands
VITAMIN B-6 (PYRIDOXINE)	2	Meats, vegetables, whole-grain cereals	Coenzyme (pyridoxal phosphate) involved in amino acid metabolism	Irritability, convulsions, muscular twitching, dermatitis near eyes, kidney stones	None reported
PANTOTHENIC ACID	5–10	Widely distributed in foods.	Constituent of coenzyme A, which plays a central role in energy metabolism	Fatigue, sleep disturbances, impaired coordination, nausea (rare in man)	None reported
FOLACIN	.4	Legumes, green vegetables, whole-wheat products	Coenzyme (reduced form) involved in transfer of single-carbon units in nucleic acid and amino acid metabolism	Anemia, gastrointestinal disturbances, diarrhea, red tongue	None reported
VITAMIN B-12	.003	Muscle meats, eggs, dairy products, (not present in plant foods)	Coenzyme involved in transfer of single-carbon units in nucleic acid metabolism	Pernicious anemia, neurological disorders	None reported
BIOTIN	Not established. Usual diet provides .15–.3	Legumes, vegetables, meats	Coenzyme required for fat synthesis, amino acid metabolism and glycogen (animal-starch) formation	Fatigue, depression, nausea, dermatitis, muscular pains	Not reported
CHOLINE	Not established. Usual diet provides 500–900	All foods containing phospholipids (egg yolk, liver, grains, legumes)	Constituent of phospholipids. Precursor of putative neurotransmitter acetylcholine	Not reported in man.	None reported
VITAMIN C (ASCORBIC ACID)	45	Citrus fruits, tomatoes, green peppers, salad greens	Maintains intercellular matrix of cartilage, bone and dentine. Important in collagen synthesis.	Scurvy (degeneration of skin, teeth, blood vessels, epithelial hemorrhages)	Relatively nontoxic. Possibility of kidney stones.
FAT-SOLUBLE					
VITAMIN A (RETINOL)	1	Provitamin A (beta-carotene) widely distributed in green vegetables. Retinol present in milk, butter, cheese, fortified margarine.	Constituent of rhodopsin (visual pigment). Maintenance of epithelial tissues. Role in mucopolysaccharide synthesis.	Xerophthalmia (keratinization of ocular tissue), night blindness, permanent blindness	Headache, vomiting, peeling of skin, anorexia, swelling of long bones
VITAMIN D	.01	Cod-liver oil, eggs, dairy products, fortified milk and margarine.	Promotes growth and mineralization of bones. Increases absorption of calcium.	Rickets (bone deformities) in children. Osteomalacia in adults.	Vomiting, diarrhea, loss of weight, kidney damage
VITAMIN E (TOCOPHEROL)	15	Seeds, green leafy vegetables, margarines, shortenings	Functions as an antitoxidant to prevent cell-membrane damage.	Possibly anemia	Relatively nontoxic
VITAMIN K (PHYLLOQUINONE)	.03	Green leafy vegetables. Small amount in cereals, fruits and meats	Important in blood clotting (involved in formation of active prothrombin)	Conditioned deficiencies associated with severe bleeding, internal hemorrhages.	Relatively nontoxic. Synthetic forms at high doses may cause jaundice.

VITAMINS are organic molecules needed in very small amounts in the diet of higher animals. Most of the water-soluble (B complex) vitamins act as coenzymes, or organic catalysts; the four fat-soluble vitamins (A, D, E and K) have more diverse functions. Although low vitamin intake can result in deficiency disease, the misguided use of high-potency vitamin pills can also have undesirable effects.

applied only to a reasonably healthy population. In spite of their limitations, however, estimates of caloric requirements and recommended allowances for essential nutrients must be supplied. They guide the design of diets for individuals, the evaluation of the relative adequacy of diets for populations, the content of nutrition-education programs and the planning by government of nutrition-intervention programs.

There is no area of human health in which research is more urgently needed than the nutritional requirements of representative human populations over the full range of both health and disease. Clearly an adequate knowledge of the amount and kinds of food required by man is essential for food and nutrition policy planning and will be of major importance for the generations ahead.

MINERAL	AMOUNT IN ADULT BODY (GRAMS)	RDA FOR HEALTHY ADULT MALE (MILLIGRAMS)	DIETARY SOURCES	MAJOR BODY FUNCTIONS	DEFICIENCY	EXCESS
CALCIUM	1,500	800	Milk, cheese, dark-green vegetables, dried legumes	Bone and tooth formation Blood clotting Nerve transmission	Stunted growth Rickets, osteoporosis Convulsions	Not reported in man
PHOSPHORUS	860	800	Milk, cheese, meat, poultry, grains	Bone and tooth formation Acid-base balance	Weakness, demineralization of bone Loss of calcium	Erosion of jaw (fossy jaw)
SULFUR	300	(Provided by sulfur amino acids)	Sulfur amino acids (methionine and cystine) in dietary proteins	Constituent of active tissue compounds, cartilage and tendon	Related to intake and deficiency of sulfur amino acids	Excess sulfur amino acid intake leads to poor growth
POTASSIUM	180	2,500	Meats, milk, many fruits	Acid-base balance Body water balance Nerve function	Muscular weakness Paralysis	Muscular weakness Death
CHLORINE	74	2,000	Common salt	Formation of gastric juice Acid-base balance	Muscle cramps Mental apathy Reduced appetite	Vomiting
SODIUM	64	2,500	Common salt	Acid-base balance Body water balance Nerve function	Muscle cramps Mental apathy Reduced appetite	High blood pressure
MAGNESIUM	25	350	Whole grains, green leafy vegetables	Activates enzymes. Involved in protein synthesis	Growth failure Behavioral disturbances Weakness, spasms	Diarrhea
IRON	4.5	10	Eggs, lean meats, legumes, whole grains, green leafy vegetables	Constituent of hemoglobin and enzymes involved in energy metabolism	Iron-deficiency anemia (weakness, reduced resistance to infection)	Siderosis Cirrhosis of liver
FLUORINE	2.6	2	Drinking water, tea, seafood	May be important in maintenance of bone structure	Higher frequency of tooth decay	Mottling of teeth Increased bone density Neurological disturbances
ZINC	2	15	Widely distributed in foods	Constituent of enzymes involved in digestion	Growth failure Small sex glands	Fever, nausea, vomiting, diarrhea
COPPER	.1	2	Meats, drinking water	Constituent of enzymes associated with iron metabolism	Anemia, bone changes (rare in man)	Rare metabolic condition (Wilson's disease)
SILICON VANADIUM TIN NICKEL	.024 .018 .017 .010	Not established	Widely distributed in foods	Function unknown (essential for animals)	Not reported in man	Industrial exposures: Silicon – silicosis Vanadium – lung irritation Tin – vomiting Nickel – acute pneumonitis
SELENIUM	.013	Not established (Diet provides .05–.1 per day)	Seafood, meat, grains	Functions in close association with vitamin E	Anemia (rare)	Gastrointestinal disorders, lung irritation
MANGANESE	.012	Not established (Diet provides 6–8 per day)	Widely distributed in foods	Constituent of enzymes involved in fat synthesis	In animals: poor growth, disturbances of nervous system, reproductive abnormalities	Poisoning in manganese mines: generalized disease of nervous system
IODINE	.011	.14	Marine fish and shellfish, dairy products, many vegetables	Constituent of thyroid hormones	Goiter (enlarged thyroid)	Very high intakes depress thyroid activity
MOLYBDENUM	.009	Not established (Diet provides .4 per day)	Legumes, cereals, organ meats	Constituent of some enzymes	Not reported in man	Inhibition of enzymes
CHROMIUM	.006	Not established (Diet provides .05–.12 per day)	Fats, vegetable oils, meats	Involved in glucose and energy metabolism	Impaired ability to metabolize glucose	Occupational exposures: skin and kidney damage
COBALT	.0015	(Required as vitamin B-12)	Organ and muscle meats, milk	Constituent of vitamin B-12	Not reported in man	Industrial exposure: dermatitis and diseases of red blood cells
WATER	40,000 (60 percent of body weight)	1.5 liters per day	Solid foods, liquids, drinking water	Transport of nutrients Temperature regulation Participates in metabolic reactions	Thirst, dehydration	Headaches, nausea Edema High blood pressure

ESSENTIAL MINERAL ELEMENTS are involved in the electrochemical functions of nerve and muscle, the formation of bones and teeth, the activation of enzymes and, in the case of iron, the transport of oxygen. The trace minerals nickel, tin, vanadium and silicon, previously considered to be health hazards, are now known to be essential for animals. Although they are so widely distributed in nature that primary dietary deficiencies are unlikely, changes in the balance among them may have important consequences for health.

4

The Cycles of
Plant and Animal Nutrition

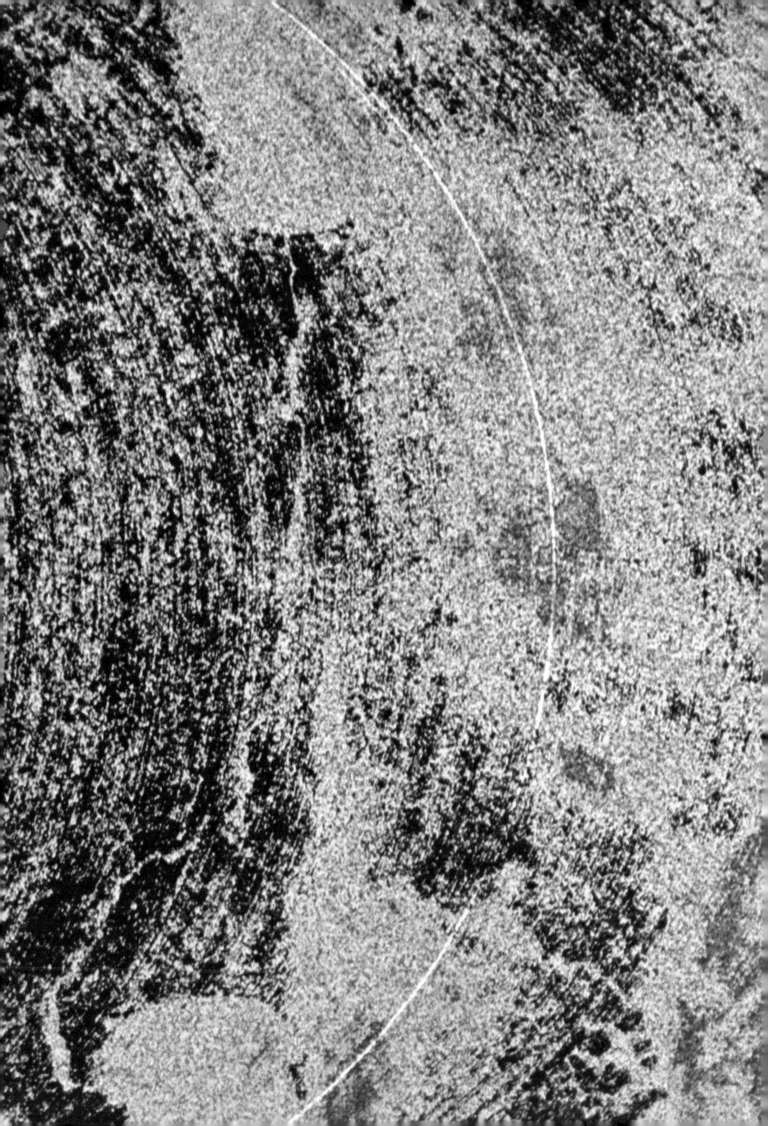

The Cycles of Plant and Animal Nutrition

JULES JANICK, CARL H. NOLLER AND CHARLES L. RHYKERD

Energy and inorganic nutrients are processed for human consumption by plants, animals and microorganisms. Modern agriculture ensures man's food supply by subsidizing the growth of these other species

The nutrition of all forms of life is necessarily in equilibrium. The solar energy absorbed by photosynthetic plants is passed along to a variety of other organisms, and it may take a long and complicated path through the biosphere. Ultimately, however, all of it is radiated back into space; if it were not, the temperature of the earth would rise. Similarly, inorganic substances in soil, water and air are absorbed by photosynthetic plants and incorporated into organic molecules that become the nutrients for animals, for certain other plants and for microorganisms. Some of these substances may be sequestered for long periods in an inaccessible form, but if the biological system is stable, all of them must eventually be returned to the pool of plant nutrients.

Because of the requirement of equilibrium the global biological system can be considered as being a continuous flow of energy and nutrients through a network of interlocking cycles. The function of agriculture is to divert this flow to the benefit of a single species. Natural forms of vegetation are replaced by cultivated varieties that have been selected for their efficiency in manufacturing foodstuff for man. Domesticated animals are introduced for a similar purpose. A third essential link in the food chain—the microorganisms—still consists mainly of wild species, but agricultural technology may eventually intervene in this part of the cycle as well.

The diversion of the flow of nutrients through the food cycle is the aim of all agricultural technologies. The distinction of modern agriculture is that it has augmented the food supply by increasing the rate at which nutrients flow through the cycle. This has been accomplished by several methods, but by far the most common and one of the most important consists in speeding the return of nutrients to the soil, where they can be reabsorbed. Hence in order to feed the human population we must ensure the nutrition of an assortment of plants, animals and microorganisms.

The earth intercepts a vast amount of solar energy, but only a little of it is available for biological purposes. About 60 percent is reflected without interacting further and most of the remainder is absorbed by the atmosphere or by oceans and landmasses and is promptly reradiated as heat. On the scale of the planetary energy budget the amount of sunlight absorbed by green plants and stored in chemical form is almost insignificant. It is less than 1 percent of the total incident energy, and it is well within the range of computational error.

In the plant, sunlight is absorbed by pigments: molecules whose bright colors signify that they strongly absorb some part of the optical spectrum. The most important pigment is chlorophyll, which absorbs both red and blue light, but several others are also found in almost all plants; together they can make use of almost all wavelengths in the visible part of the spectrum.

The solar energy absorbed is employed by the plant to drive a complicated sequence of chemical reactions that has the net effect of transferring two atoms of hydrogen from a molecule of water to a molecule of carbon dioxide. The products of the reaction are free

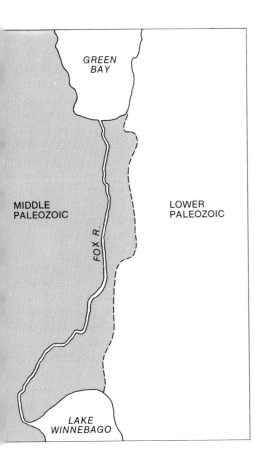

GREEN BAY

MIDDLE PALEOZOIC

LOWER PALEOZOIC

FOX R.

LAKE WINNEBAGO

ENERGY EQUILIBRIUM of the earth's surface is suggested by the image on the opposite page, made with radiation in the thermal infrared portion of the electromagnetic spectrum. The photograph was made in August, 1973, from an altitude of 275 miles by an instrument on *Skylab 3.* It covers the region in the vicinity of Green Bay, Wis., shown in the map at the left. The intensity of the thermal infrared radiation emitted by a surface is determined mainly by its temperature. Here the relative level of emissions is indicated by color; in order of increasing intensity the colors are white, cyan, red, green, blue, yellow, magenta and black. The broad belt of land that appears mainly yellow and magenta borders on Lake Michigan, which is just beyond the frame of the image to the right. Yellow and magenta also predominate in Lake Winnebago and Green Bay. The most distinctive feature of the landscape is an abrupt transition to stronger thermal emissions, which appear black. The transition corresponds to a boundary between regions of different underlying geology and different topography. The yellow-and-magenta area is mainly wet lowlands; the black area is more hilly and somewhat drier. The entire region is one of intense agricultural development, being given over mainly to dairy farms. All the solar energy absorbed by the earth is eventually reradiated into space, much of it at thermal infrared wavelengths. The small part employed by plants for photosynthesis passes through food chain before being reradiated.

44

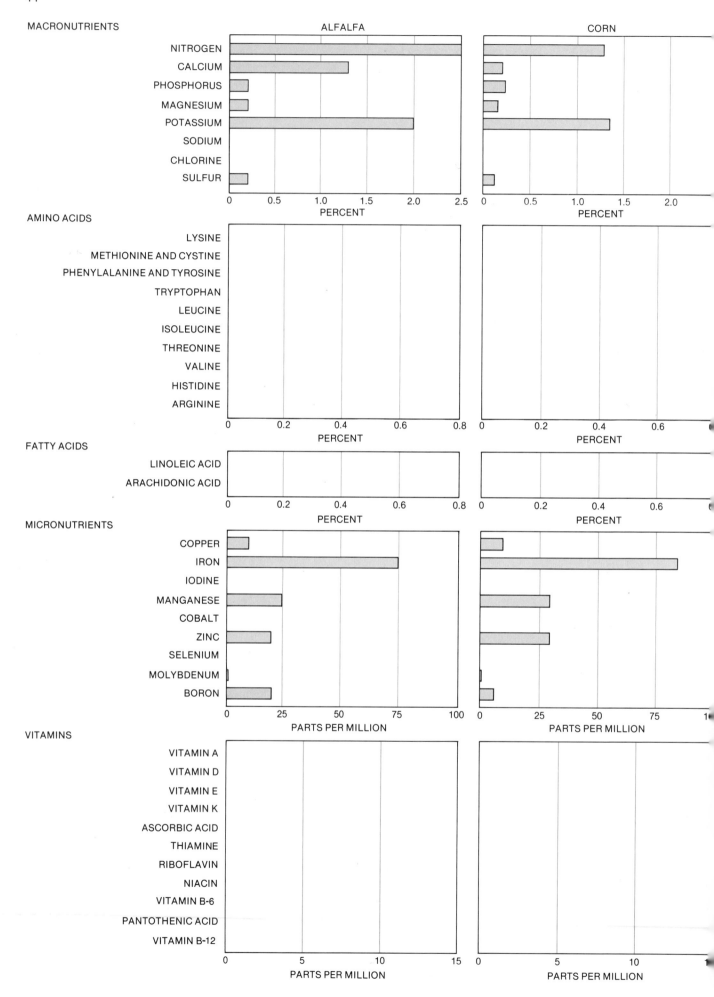

MACRONUTRIENTS

ALFALFA

CORN

NITROGEN
CALCIUM
PHOSPHORUS
MAGNESIUM
POTASSIUM
SODIUM
CHLORINE
SULFUR

PERCENT

PERCENT

AMINO ACIDS

LYSINE
METHIONINE AND CYSTINE
PHENYLALANINE AND TYROSINE
TRYPTOPHAN
LEUCINE
ISOLEUCINE
THREONINE
VALINE
HISTIDINE
ARGININE

PERCENT

PERCENT

FATTY ACIDS

LINOLEIC ACID
ARACHIDONIC ACID

PERCENT

PERCENT

MICRONUTRIENTS

COPPER
IRON
IODINE
MANGANESE
COBALT
ZINC
SELENIUM
MOLYBDENUM
BORON

PARTS PER MILLION

PARTS PER MILLION

VITAMINS

VITAMIN A
VITAMIN D
VITAMIN E
VITAMIN K
ASCORBIC ACID
THIAMINE
RIBOFLAVIN
NIACIN
VITAMIN B-6
PANTOTHENIC ACID
VITAMIN B-12

PARTS PER MILLION

PARTS PER MILLION

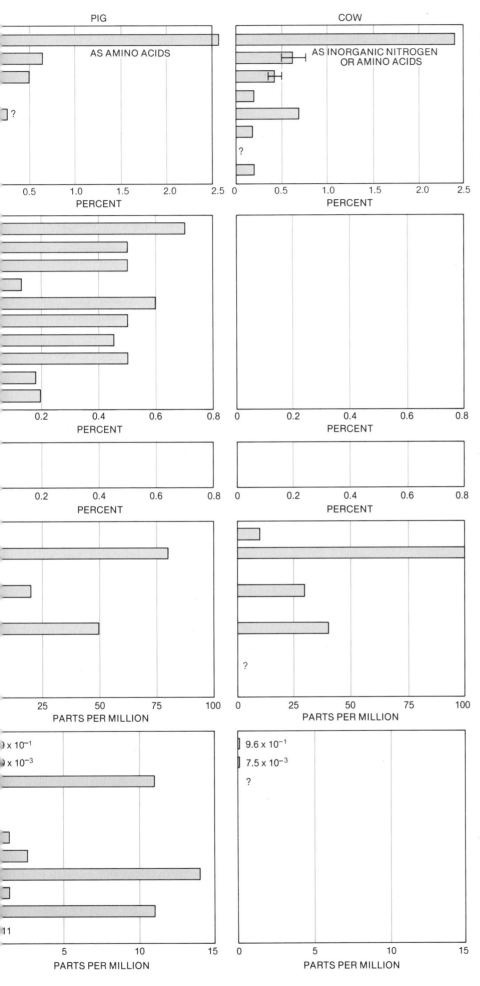

oxygen, which is released to the atmosphere, and carbohydrates, compounds made up of carbon, hydrogen and oxygen. The energy of these products is greater than that of the carbon dioxide and the water; the added energy can be recovered and put to work. It can be recovered most simply by recombining the oxygen and the carbohydrates; that process, respiration, is the principal mechanism from which the vast majority of organisms derive their energy.

Carbon that has been converted to organic form through photosynthesis is called fixed carbon. Some of it is utilized immediately to meet the metabolic needs of the plant, including the synthesis of other essential molecules, such as the amino acids that make up proteins. The rest of the fixed carbon is stored, usually in the form of polysaccharides: large molecules made of many simple sugar units linked together. By far the commonest polysaccharide in plants is cellulose, the fibrous material responsible for the rigidity and structural integrity of leaves and stems. Energy reserves for the plant and its progeny are often provided by another polysaccharide, starch, stored in seeds and in specialized organs such as tubers, rhizomes, bulbs and corms. Animals derive almost all their energy directly or indirectly from the decomposition of these two polysaccharides. Cellulose and starch are closely related: both consist of long chains of the sugar glucose. They differ only in the geometry of the bonds between the glucose units. This small difference in structure, however, brings vast differences in the physical properties of the two molecules and in their suitability as a constituent of animal diets.

Green plants capture solar energy with an efficiency of from 15 to 22 percent, which exceeds the efficiency of energy conversion in many industrial technologies. The energy represented by the fixed carbon is passed along the food chain when plant materials are consumed by other organisms. With each transition a portion of the energy is lost, in some cases the major portion. A hundred thousand pounds of marine algae must be transferred through the food chain to produce a pound of codfish. All the remaining energy of the algae is dissipated, mainly as heat. The codfish it-

NUTRITIONAL NEEDS of plants and animals are fundamentally different. The nutritional needs of plants can be expressed as a list of elements, whereas animals require more complex, organic molecules, such as amino acids (the constituents of proteins), fatty acids and vitamins in addition to minerals. Among animals the ruminants are exceptional in that many of their nutritional requirements can be met through the synthetic activities of microorganisms in the rumen. In addition to the nutrients shown, all organisms require carbon, hydrogen and oxygen.

self is soon reduced to heat and a few low-energy substances: carbon dioxide, water and minerals.

This enormous loss of energy may seem improvident, but it is not germane to the problem of feeding the human population. The annual production of fixed carbon by green plants on land and in the seas is about 150 billion tons; human consumption is about 260 pounds per person. Thus the energy captured by plants far exceeds human needs; if it could all be directed to human nutrition, it could support a population of 1.15 trillion, more than 280 times the present population. The food supply is not limited by a scarcity of sunshine.

The quantity of energy that is important in calculations of agricultural efficiency is the energy that must be supplied by man in order to concentrate and extract nutrients. Under natural conditions plant life is often sparsely distributed and little of the available organic matter is in a form directly useful to man. The intermediary use of a grazing steer is an inefficient step in the conversion of sunlight to human food. On rangeland, however, where the available plant life is scattered and consists mainly of grasses and other species with a high fiber content, the steer harvests the nutrients under its own power, with

only a small energy subsidy from man. Most of the final product—beefsteak—represents a net gain.

Few habitats are so harsh that nothing will grow: the arctic and alpine regions have their tiny wildflowers, and even the urban sidewalk is pierced by crabgrass. Under such circumstances plants make effective use of very scarce nutrients. Agriculture is profitable, however, only where a plant species of some value to man can be grown with a high yield. If a worthwhile yield is to be achieved, all the nutrients needed by the plant must be supplied in virtually optimum amounts.

Compared with the complex nutritional requirements of man and of other animals the needs of plants are quite simple. Plants subsist entirely on inorganic materials, and even they make up only a short list. The major nutrients are carbon dioxide, oxygen and water, and these substances are required in quantities so large that they are often considered in a category apart from the other nutrients. Carbon dioxide and oxygen are of course universally available (at least to land plants), and under field conditions they probably never fall to levels low enough to impair growth. Water is also an abundant resource, although it is

less uniformly distributed. The relation of water supply to plant growth has surely been understood since before the beginnings of agriculture. Water is often a factor limiting growth, and the correction of water deficiency by irrigation can yield spectacular benefits.

In all, 16 elements are known to be necessary for the growth of plants. Air and water supply carbon, hydrogen and oxygen. In addition to these three elements, nitrogen, potassium and calcium are required in relatively large quantities. The remaining nutrients are needed in lesser amounts, and for some only a trace is needed. They are phosphorus, magnesium, sulfur, manganese, boron, iron, zinc, copper, molybdenum and chlorine.

Except for carbon, hydrogen and oxygen, all the nutrients must be absorbed from the soil. The nutrition of plants is thus dependent on the ability of the soil to store essential elements and to make them available in a biologically active form. Many of the most important events in the growth of a crop take place below the surface of the soil; as a result soil occupies a central position in several biological cycles.

Soil is formed by the weathering and disintegration of rock and by the synthesis of both crystalline and amorphous minerals. In addition, the character and composition of the soil are altered by biological activity. The process of soil formation is a continuous, evolutionary one. Vertical sections of most soils reveal a sequence of horizons, or layers: at the surface there may be a layer of loose litter, below that a layer rich in organic material and often called "topsoil," below that the "subsoil" and finally the parent rock in various stages of weathering. The soil profile is a historical document, recording the sequence of processes that contributed to the development of the soil.

The mineral components of soil are classified according to the size of their particles as clay, silt, sand and gravel. In addition there is an important organic constituent, humus, that is made up of decay-resistant residues such as lignins, waxes, fats and some proteinaceous materials. Humus has a profound influence on the physical and chemical properties of the soil. The coarser particles of silt, sand and gravel have properties essentially like those of the rock from which they are derived. Clay and humus, however, are colloids, or suspensions of microscopically fine particles, and they are the most active components of the soil. They are particularly well adapted to the retention of mineral nutrients.

The texture and structure of a soil are important in determining its suitability for agriculture. Texture is mainly a function of particle size, which in turn determines the size of the voids between particles. Sandy soils have large pores, with the result that water tends to drain

HORIZON	
0	LITTER
A	ORGANIC AND MINERAL PARTICLES
B	FINE PARTICLES
C	WEATHERED ROCK
D	ROCK

SOIL is the principal source of nutrients for plants and the site of a number of important transformations in the food cycle. The inorganic constituents of soil, produced by the weathering of rock and by the crystallization of minerals, are classified by texture as clay, silt, sand and gravel. An additional component of great importance is the organic material called humus. Clay and humus are colloids whose particles have a large surface area; they readily adsorb nutrients and retain them for later absorption by roots. A cross section of soil generally reveals a sequence of layers, or horizons; the A horizon corresponds to what is commonly called topsoil.

through them quickly; the water itself is thereby lost to roots, and it also carries away soluble nutrients. The very small pores of clay soils retain water by capillary action, providing the aqueous medium that is essential for the transport of nutrients. On the other hand, soils with too much clay can become permanently waterlogged, blocking the aeration of the roots.

The most productive soils have a crumbly structure developed when small colloidal particles are cemented together by organic materials, particularly the exudates of microorganisms. Such soils are well aerated and have a large capacity for retaining water.

The great importance of the colloidal particles of clay and humus is their capacity for adsorbing ions. The colloids have an enormous surface area with respect to their volume: in clay the surface area may reach 800 square meters per gram. Moreover, the particles bear a negative electric charge and therefore attract cations, or positively charged ions, to their surface. In this way nutrients that otherwise would be lost by leaching are held in reserve for later use by plants.

The cations are not rigidly bound to the colloidal particles, and they can be displaced by other ions. If all the ions are present in equal concentration, sodium ions are replaced by potassium ions, and they in turn are replaced by magnesium. Calcium ions replace the magnesium, and finally hydrogen ions replace the calcium. Hydrogen ions are evolved continuously as carbon dioxide dissolves in the groundwater and forms carbonic acid; the carbon dioxide is released by the respiration of living roots and by the biological decay of carbohydrates. The steady release of hydrogen ions promotes the exchange of cations, making them available for plant growth. The supply of the other cations is replenished by the decomposition of rock and the degradation of organic materials. In an agricultural context, of course, the concentrations of all the cations can be altered at will by the application of fertilizers, but the importance of clay and humus in storing the nutrients and making them available to roots remains.

The cation-exchange capacity of a soil depends on the amount of humus and clay present and on the composition of the clay. Sand is relatively inert, and sandy soils low in organic matter are unreactive and infertile, although they can be made productive by fertilization and irrigation. Silt is slightly more reactive than sand but is generally much less reactive than clay. Clays differ in their ability to exchange cations by a factor of 10; humus may be twice as reactive as the most reactive clays. For this reason humus plays a role in plant nutrition out of proportion to the modest amounts of it found in most soils.

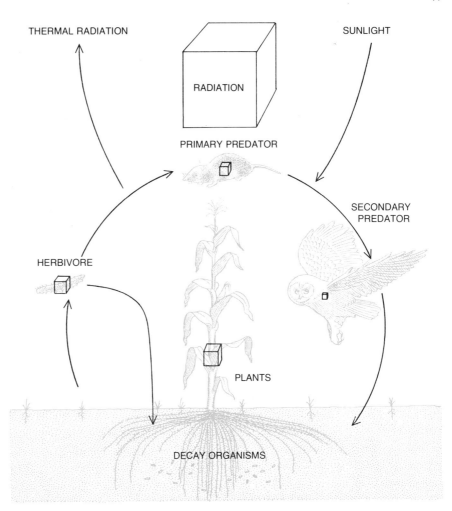

ENERGY CYCLE in the biosphere is driven by the photosynthetic activities of green plants. The plants employ solar energy to convert inorganic nutrients into energy-rich organic compounds, particularly carbohydrates and proteins. Almost all other organisms sustain life by breaking down the products of photosynthesis into their simpler constituents. All animals, for example, depend for their nutrition entirely on plant life, directly in the case of herbivores, indirectly in the case of primary and secondary predators. Finally, the waste products and dead tissues of both plants and animals make up the diet of decay organisms, which extract the remaining available energy from these materials and return them to inorganic form. The relative quantities of radiant energy received by the earth and radiated back into space and the biomass of the various organisms in the food chain are represented by the volume of the cubes.

In the humid Tropics soils tend to be of low productivity: their clays have a low capacity for cation exchange and humus does not accumulate because the high temperatures of equatorial climates promote the rapid decomposition of organic matter. The problem is exacerbated by copious precipitation, which leaches nutrients from the soil. The lush vegetation of the humid Tropics seems to suggest great agricultural potential; actually the fertility of the soil is low. The plants of the rain forest are able to achieve their luxuriant growth only because they are adapted to their habitat and rapidly absorb the nutrients released by decaying organic matter before they can be leached away. This equilibrium is fragile. The direct extension of the agricultural practices of the Temperate Zone to tropical climates is seldom successful because the nutrient cycle is broken and productivity steadily declines.

The pH of the soil has a profound effect on plant growth. Abnormally alkaline soils (those with a pH of 9 or above) and very acid soils (with a pH of 4 or below) are in themselves toxic to roots. Between these extremes the direct effect of soil pH on most plants is minor, but the indirect effect on the availability of nutrients can be tremendous. Phosphorus, for example, becomes insoluble and therefore unavailable if the soil is either very acid or very alkaline. The pH also affects soil organisms, particularly bacteria. High acidity, which is typical of humid areas, inhibits both nitrogen fixation and the decay process. Acid soils can be neutralized by applying limestone (ground calcium carbonate and magnesium carbonate rock); excessive alkalinity, which is typical of arid areas, can be corrected by the addition of acid-forming fertilizers or by leaching to remove excess salts.

A final component of soil that must not be neglected is the indigenous population of living organisms. An acre-foot

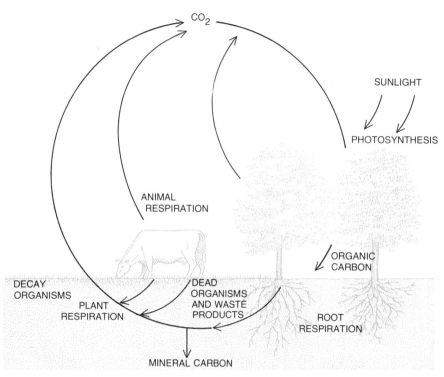

CARBON CYCLE involves two competing processes: photosynthesis and respiration. During photosynthesis plants convert carbon dioxide and water into carbohydrates and free oxygen. The latter combination of substances represents a rich store of energy, which is utilized in respiration as the carbohydrates and oxygen are recombined to yield carbon dioxide and water again. Respiration is common to all organisms that can live in the presence of oxygen, and thus all contribute to the return of carbon dioxide to the atmosphere. Some carbon is sequestered in minerals such as coal and petroleum, but that too is returned to the cycle when it is burned.

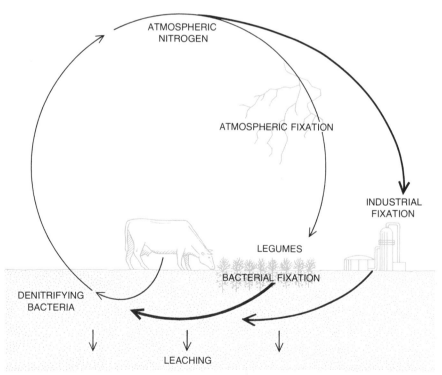

NITROGEN CYCLE traces the circulation of the nutrient that is often the factor limiting the growth of plants. Atmospheric nitrogen is useless to plants; the element must be supplied in "fixed," or combined, form, as in ammonium ions (NH_4^+) or nitrate ions (NO_3^-). A little nitrogen is fixed by lightning and other processes in the atmosphere, and a more important contribution is made by bacteria, notably those that live symbiotically in the root nodules of legumes. Nevertheless, the pool of available nitrogen in most soils remains small. The element is removed by leaching and by bacteria that return it to the atmosphere, and it is lost through the harvesting of crops. To compensate for these losses nitrogen fixed industrially is applied to the soil as fertilizer; industrial fixation has become a major component of the nitrogen cycle.

of fertile soil may contain more than three tons of living matter, including bacteria, fungi, protozoa, algae, nematodes, worms and insects. These organisms are entirely responsible for the breakdown of organic matter into simple nutrients that can be absorbed by plant roots. The microorganisms feed on plant and animal refuse and the plants feed on the excretions and decay products of the microorganisms. Soil fauna and microorganisms also help to maintain soil structure and aeration.

In the mid-19th century Justus von Liebig formulated his law of the minimum, which states that plant growth is limited by the availability of whatever nutrient is scarcest. Thus it is of little benefit to irrigate a crop that is stunted for lack of nitrogen, and if the nitrogen deficiency is corrected, some other nutrient will become the limiting factor. The strategy of agriculture must be to provide all nutrients in adequate amounts and in optimum proportions.

Nitrogen is commonly the limiting element. Because it is a constituent of all proteins and of many other biological molecules it is required in relatively large amounts. Furthermore, much nitrogen is removed from the soil by leaching and erosion, by the action of microorganisms and by the plants themselves. The amount readily available in most soils is small.

Nitrogen, of course, is the major constituent of the atmosphere, and the column of air above an acre of land contains 75 million pounds of it. This form of nitrogen, however, is useless to most plants; to be biologically active the nitrogen must be "fixed" by being combined with other elements. In nature nitrogen fixation is accomplished in the soil, primarily by bacteria. The most efficient of these bacteria are symbiotic: they fix nitrogen only in association with the roots of legumes and of some tropical grasses.

Nitrogen in the soil is found largely in organic matter in various stages of decomposition, but the nitrogen remains unavailable to plants until it is converted to ammonium ions (NH_4^+) or nitrate (NO_3^-) ions. The circuitous route of nitrogen from element to amino acid to protein and back to the elemental form is the most intensely studied of the nutrient cycles. Much of plant and animal nutrition pivots on the availability of nitrogen-containing compounds.

The breakdown of proteins into amino acids in the soil is carried out by bacteria, which utilize the energy released by this process for their own growth. Only after the death and disintegration of the bacteria is the nitrogen available to roots.

The further breakdown of amino acids into inorganic nitrogen compounds is accomplished in several steps, each mediated by a specific group of bacteria.

First, ammonium ions are liberated from the amino acids; then the ammonium ions are converted to nitrite ions (NO_2^-) and finally to nitrate ions (NO_3^-). The bacteria that produce nitrites and nitrates are autotrophic and aerobic, that is, they do not require organic nutrition but do require oxygen. They are greatly affected by soil aeration and by temperature and moisture.

Like the conversion of nitrogen to a form in which it can be assimilated, the removal of nitrogen from the soil is largely a biological process. Much of it is lost to plants, and when a crop is harvested, the loss is permanent. Fixed nitrogen is also removed from the pool of nutrients by certain soil bacteria, which convert nitrates back to atmospheric nitrogen. This process is an anaerobic one: it can proceed only in the absence of oxygen. Thus a lack of proper aeration results in the loss of available nitrogen. Furthermore, nitrates are readily soluble in water, and if they are not utilized by microorganisms or higher plants, they can be lost by leaching. The level of available nitrogen is therefore dependent on the amount of organic matter in the soil, on the population of microorganisms and on the extent of leaching.

Under natural, nonagricultural conditions an equilibrium is reached between the rate of plant growth and the forces that affect the supply of nitrogen in the soil. In many agricultural systems, however, this equilibrium is disturbed. The harvesting of a crop tends to deplete nitrogen not only through the direct effects of removing the plant life but also through increased erosion and a reduction in soil organic matter. For this reason intensive agriculture depends on the addition of nitrogen as fertilizer.

Traditionally nitrogen fertilizers were derived from organic sources, particularly animal manures such as guano: the accumulated droppings of birds. Later supplies included sodium nitrate, mined in Chile, and ammonium sulfate, a byproduct of coke ovens. Today most nitrogen fertilizer is synthesized by the Haber process, in which atmospheric nitrogen is reacted with hydrogen to form ammonia. The ammonia can be applied directly or it can be employed as a raw material for the manufacture of urea, nitrates or other nitrogen compounds.

The hydrogen required by the Haber process is generally extracted from natural gas, and the cost of that fuel makes up most of the cost of the manufactured nitrogen fertilizer. The synthesis of a ton of anhydrous ammonia requires 30,000 cubic feet of natural gas. Hence through industrial nitrogen fixation fossil fuels enter directly into the nutrient cycle; their cost is recouped through the value added to the crop by fertilization.

The remaining nutrient elements are somewhat less likely to present a limitation to growth, but that is not to say they are less important. In some cases

the amount required is small, but it is an absolute requirement. Phosphorus is a constituent of nucleic acids and of several molecules involved in the transport of energy, but it is required only in small amounts. Dry plant materials contain about 2 percent nitrogen but only .2 percent phosphorus. Nevertheless, most soils are unable to supply enough phosphorus for maximum growth. Phosphorus, unlike nitrogen, is relatively stable in the soil and leaching is negligible; on the other hand, the availability of phosphorus is dependent on soil *p*H. Phosphate fertilizer is widely applied, most often in the form of "superphosphates" obtained by treating rock phosphate with sulfuric acid or phosphoric acid.

Potassium is required in relatively large amounts, although its precise role

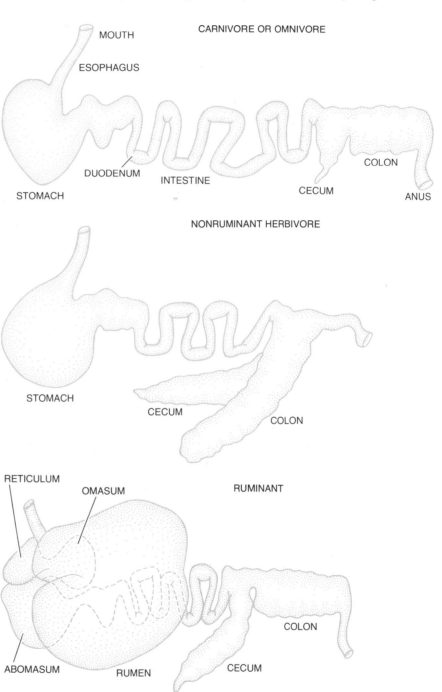

ANATOMY OF THE DIGESTIVE TRACT is the principal determinant of animal diet; in particular it determines whether or not an animal can derive sustenance from cellulose, the most abundant plant product. The digestion of cellulose is dependent on enzymes secreted by bacteria. In animals with simple stomachs, including carnivores such as the dog and omnivores such as man and the pig, the appropriate bacteria are found only in the cecum and colon, and the food passes through these structures too quickly for digestion to be effective. In nonruminant herbivores such as the horse the cecum and colon are more highly developed, but residence time is still limited and some nutrients required by the bacteria are removed earlier in the tract, so that cellulose digestion is inefficient. In ruminants, such as the cow, the bacterial degradation of cellulose is accomplished at the start of the alimentary tract, in the rumen. The full length of the intestine, cecum and colon is available for the absorption of the nutrients.

in plant physiology is not well understood. It is available as an exchangeable ion adsorbed on the soil colloid. Soils that contain relatively little humus are often rich in potassium, but it is in an insoluble form and therefore unavailable. Organic soils are usually deficient in potassium. Hence fertilization is often required; the major fertilizer is potassium chloride.

The calcium content of plants varies by species (it is low in grasses and high in legumes), but calcium is seldom deficient as a nutrient. The collateral effects of calcium on the soil, however, are numerous, with the result that the calcium content is frequently amended. The element has an influence on the activities of microorganisms, on pH and on the absorption of other ions. Calcium is present in the soil as a water-soluble, exchangeable cation, in combination with organic compounds and in insoluble minerals such as the feldspars hornblende and calcite.

Magnesium, a constituent of the chlorophyll molecule, is absorbed by roots as an ion. It is found in the soil solution as an exchangeable cation, and deficiencies are rare.

Sulfur, a constituent of two amino acids, cystine and methionine, and of the vitamins biotin and thiamine, is not available in large amounts in the soil. It is continually leached, but new supplies are also continuously added by the breakdown of sulfur-containing minerals, such as pyrite. In industrial regions sulfur is also added by rainfall, since rain absorbs sulfur dioxide from industrial pollution.

Manganese, boron, iron, zinc, copper, molybdenum and chlorine are required by plants only in minute amounts. Deficiencies, although not widespread, can severely limit productivity. Molybdenum deficiency has been implicated as a factor causing low levels of nitrogen fixation in some areas.

Apart from light, air and water, the most conspicuous demand a plant makes on its environment is for minerals. Animals too require minerals, but they also have more complex dietary needs, which cannot be expressed by a simple list of chemical elements. The nourishment of animals is dependent on organic substances: carbohydrates, fats, vitamins and proteins or the amino acids of which proteins are made. All these substances must be derived directly or indirectly from green plants, and animals are therefore effectively parasites on the plant community. They obtain energy by breaking down the energy-rich products of photosynthesis into simpler, less energetic molecules. For example, an animal can ingest glucose and combine it with oxygen to release energy, carbon dioxide and water; this process, respiration, is the exact opposite of photosynthesis.

Virtually all animals feed in essential-ly the same way: organic substances are ingested and partially decomposed by digestive enzymes so that the nutrients can be absorbed. The partial decomposition is the function of the digestive tract. The species differ, however, in the kinds of food that are acceptable to them. Among the vertebrates the most significant distinction is between those animals that gain sustenance from cellulose and those that require other forms of carbohydrate.

The importance of this distinction reflects the extraordinary importance of cellulose in the global nutrient cycle. A major share of the energy budget of most green plants is dedicated to the manufacture of cellulose, and cellulose is the most abundant material in the structure of plants. It represents an enormous energy resource.

Mammals do not make enzymes that are capable of breaking the bonds between the glucose units in cellulose, and it therefore has no direct nutritive value for them. A number of bacteria do secrete the appropriate enzymes. Mammals that sustain themselves on a diet rich in cellulose are able to do so by virtue of the fact that these bacteria grow in their digestive tract. Through fermentation the bacteria partially decompose the cellulose, skimming off some of the energy to support their own life cycle. The decomposition is completed by the host animal, which by reducing the molecules to carbon dioxide and water extracts the remaining energy. Moreover, the dead bacteria can also be digested. The dietary strategy amounts to a kind of internal agriculture.

Animals can be classified in three groups based on their abilities to assimilate cellulose, a classification that is reflected in the structure of their digestive apparatus. Carnivores, such as the dog, and omnivores, such as man and the pig, have simple stomachs and have difficulty digesting cellulose. Nonruminant herbivores, such as the horse, the rabbit and the guinea pig, can derive sustenance from cellulose, but they assimilate it less efficiently than the ruminants. Ruminant herbivores, such as cattle, sheep, goats, deer, buffalo and many others, can efficiently break down cellulose and extract a large proportion of their dietary calories from it.

In animals with simple stomachs digestion is carried out mainly by indigenous enzymes: those secreted by the animal itself. Most of the enzymes are manufactured in the pancreas and by mucosal cells in the wall of the stomach and the small intestine. The main site of nutrient absorption is the small intestine. Bacteria are found in the cecum and colon, but food residues pass through these parts of the digestive tract quickly, with little bacterial digestion.

In nonruminant herbivores the bacte-rial populations of the cecum and colon are more important. Dietary cellulose is digested there by the bacteria, producing acetic acid, propionic acid and butyric acid; these organic acids are waste products of the microorganisms but energy-rich foods for the host animal. Some of the amino acids and vitamins

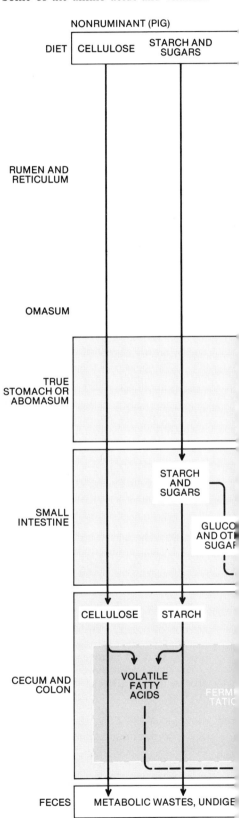

DIETARY STRATEGY of ruminants and nonruminants differs markedly. Nonruminants simply assimilate that portion of their

synthesized by the bacteria can also be absorbed.

The efficiency of this process may be limited because some nutrients required by the bacteria are absorbed in the small intestine, before they reach the microorganisms. Moreover, some of the nutritionally valuable products of the bacte-

ria may be lost in the feces because of inefficient absorption in the cecum and colon.

The superlative adaptation to the challenge of a diet rich in cellulose is found in the ruminants. Bacterial fermentation of fibrous foods is concentrated in an extensive fermentation vat,

the rumen, at the beginning of the digestive tract. There cellulose is broken down into smaller molecules, and the capabilities of the bacteria for synthesizing amino acids and certain vitamins are exploited. The bacterial transformation is accomplished before the food enters the small intestine, so that the full

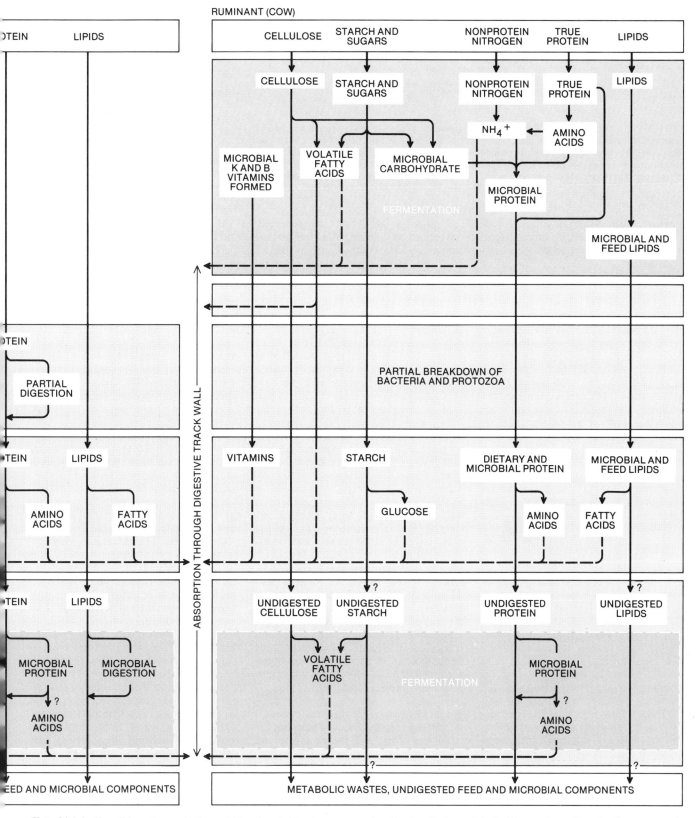

diet which is digestible and excrete the rest. Ruminants divert a portion of their food in order to raise an internal crop of bacteria. Both the waste products and the breakdown products of the bacteria can **then be absorbed as nutrients. The ruminant digestion is not more efficient than that of the nonruminant, but by breaking down cellulose it makes use of a food that otherwise would not be available at all.**

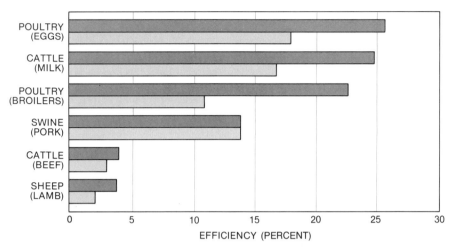

EFFICIENCY OF LIVESTOCK measures the percentage of dietary crude protein and energy converted to products edible by man. The highest efficiencies in the conversion of both protein (*gray bars*) and energy (*color*) are found in the production of eggs and milk. Cattle and sheep raised for slaughter have a low efficiency, but because their diets can be composed largely of material that is inedible to man their production can result in a net gain for human nutrition.

length of the intestine is available for the absorption of nutrients extracted from the food and synthesized by the microorganisms.

Farm animals have traditionally been sustained by the direct consumption of plant materials, such as grains and grasses, but many other nutritive materials are potential dietary resources. For example, the meal produced from soybeans, cottonseed and peanuts as a byproduct of oil extraction, and the wheat bran, beet pulp and molasses produced as a by-product of carbohydrate extraction, are all suitable feeds for many animals. Slaughterhouse wastes, such as blood, bone meal and offal, and even animal wastes, such as the manures of cattle and poultry, can be fed to cattle. Because of the ability of rumen bacteria to synthesize amino acids cattle can even be fed sources of inorganic nitrogen, such as ammonia or urea.

With the variety of feedstuffs available, the number of potential animal-ration formulations is almost unlimited. In poor countries livestock and man are in competition for the available grain. As a result grain is fed only to animals that are efficient converters of calories to tissue, such as the chicken and the pig, and to animals needed for work. Ruminants either graze or consume wastes.

In rich and agriculturally productive countries, on the other hand, there is only limited competition for food. It is therefore possible to increase the productivity of animals by supplementing their diet with grain. Swine and poultry can consume essentially all their nutrients in concentrated form. In the U.S. beef breeding cows spend almost their entire life on pasture with little or no grain, but their offspring destined for slaughter generally receive a generous portion of grain in a feedlot to increase their rate of weight gain and to improve their carcass characteristics.

Productive dairy cows are generally fed rations containing from 20 to 50 percent grain. Dairy cattle can grow, maintain themselves, reproduce and remain healthy when fed entirely on forages. On a forage of average quality, however, cows have difficulty obtaining sufficient nutrients to produce more than 10 to 20 pounds of milk per day. High-quality forages can support from 30 to 40 pounds of milk per day. With liberal grain feeding, dairy cows can produce more than 100 pounds of milk per day.

Nonruminant animals require a diet that in many respects does not differ much from the human diet. In the event of a food shortage it would theoretically be more efficient to bypass the animal and reserve the available food for human consumption. Animals, however, offer a way of refining unpalatable or inedible products and storing them in useful forms. Of the solar energy transformed into chemical energy by the plant only about 20 percent can be directly utilized by man. Animals convert plant products into human food with an efficiency that varies between 2 and 18 percent. That inefficient conversion, however, is not a loss but a gain if the photosynthetic energy consumed by the animals could not have been recovered otherwise. The justification for animals in agriculture is their ability to transform products of little or no value into nutritious human food.

In an undisturbed ecological system a balance is soon achieved between the resources of the soil, the plant life and all the organisms that feed on the plants. The biomass, or total amount of biological material that can be supported, is determined by a combination of environmental factors, of which climate is the most important. In primitive agricultural systems the natural flora and fauna are merely replaced by crops and

domesticated animals. The interaction of plants and animals may be altered only slightly; any change in the total biomass is probably small and could be either a gain or a loss. The economic impact, however, is enormous, because a much larger proportion of the biomass is of use to man.

Primitive agriculture is characterized by a small energy subsidy, low output and high overall efficiency. Animals consume excess feed, roughage and waste products; wastes from plant decay, and from animals and people, are utilized or recycled back to the soil. Power requirements are met through the labor of men, women and animals. Little is added to the system in fuel, machinery, fertilizer or pesticide, but little is removed in food in spite of unrelenting toil. Properly managed, the system is at best self-sustaining; mismanagement, either by overgrazing or by cultivation practices that lead to excessive erosion, destroys the system.

Modern agricultural systems emphasize high production and labor efficiency. The natural plant and animal cycles, the mainstay of primitive agriculture, are modified to fit a technology in which a large energy subsidy is possible. This subsidy often takes the form of manufactured goods: machinery, gasoline, fertilizer, pesticide. For maximum efficiency, production of particular crops is geographically concentrated and farms become specialized. Animals and plants are raised in widely separated places. These changes represent the response of farmers to a combination of economic forces involving climate, the concentration of population, land values, the low cost of energy and the high cost of labor. The preferences of consumers have also had a strong influence. In the U.S. it is the demand for tender cuts of beef combined with the relatively low cost of grain that makes the feeding of high-energy grains to cattle feasible.

Liebig's law of the minimum need not be confined in its application to plant nutrients; it can be extended to cover all the factors that bear on the success of the agricultural enterprise. Indeed, the history of agricultural technology has been a search for economic ways of overcoming factors that limit production. Some of the most productive lands were once worthless because they were too dry; similarly, in many parts of the world today a lack of investment capital has proved to be just as effective in limiting production as a lack of water. On the whole the success of technology in increasing agricultural productivity has been remarkable. The alarming graph of world population increase is also the reassuring graph of increasing world food production.

For additional improvements in yield many of the most promising opportunities involve intervention in the cycles that connect plants, soil, animals and microorganisms. For example, there is the potential for a large increase in the biological fixation of nitrogen. The legume alfalfa has been grown with annual yields of 16 tons per acre without the application of nitrogen fertilizers. In alfalfa containing 3 percent nitrogen the bacteria associated with the plant roots must fix at least 1,000 pounds of nitrogen per acre per year, which is five times the amount generally accepted as being typical. Nitrogen fixation in the soil might be further improved by artificially selecting efficient strains of symbiotic bacteria, coupled with more widespread adoption of improved legumes, particularly in the Tropics. It was recently discovered that bacteria capable of nitrogen fixation live in a partial symbiotic association with certain tropical grasses, including maize. The genetic manipulation of bacteria offers hope that the capacity to fix nitrogen may eventually be conferred on all crops. A development with a more immediate prospect of application is the discovery of an inexpensive substance (nitropyrin) that retards the bacterial conversion of ammonia to nitrite in the soil. Since ammonia is a cation and is retained by soil colloids, whereas nitrite and nitrate are readily leached away, nitropyrin could retard the loss of nitrogen from the soil. Finally, the absorptive capacity of some plant roots is increased by an intimate association, called mycorrhiza, between the roots and a fungus. The encouragement of mycorrhizal associations might benefit certain crop plants, particularly in infertile soils and where specific nutrients are low in availability.

A number of potential improvements in the agricultural efficiency of industrial societies are merely a matter of thrift. Many residues that are now burned or discarded could be returned to the soil to improve fertility; better still, they could be processed through animals to produce food. Organic wastes such as sewage sludge, cannery by-products and animal manures are rich sources of plant nutrients. About 44 percent of the live weight of cattle slaughtered for meat is inedible to man but is of high nutritional value as a protein concentrate for animal feeding. Nutrients are also wasted in the discarded by-products of grain milling, oil extraction, fish processing and fermentation. Billions of tons of crop residues, including straw, sugarcane refuse and sawdust, are potential feed for ruminants. In the U.S. alone 60 million acres of corn are grown for grain, which contains only half of the plant's potential energy; the other half, contained in the stalks and cobs, could be fed to animals. So could poultry and cattle manures; in fact, they are already being included in ruminant diets. The greater use of such bulky residues and by-products is limited mainly by the high cost of transportation. One possible strategy for avoiding those costs would be to decentralize animal agriculture in the U.S.

Competition for protein suitable for human consumption could be reduced and perhaps eliminated in ruminants by replacing protein in the ruminant diet with other sources of nitrogen. A lactating cow on a diet of waste roughage and urea produces more protein than it consumes. Rumen efficiency might be enhanced by rumen stimulants and digestive aids. Even nitrogen fixation has been demonstrated in the bacteria of the ruminant digestive tract and might someday be exploited.

Although man has become a manipulator of the food cycle, he is made of flesh and must still remain a participant in the cycle. A viable system of food production requires an efficient transfer of energy and exchange of nutrients between soil, plant, animal and microorganism. The relationship can be exploited for short-term gains or managed for long-term sustenance. It can be ignored only at our peril.

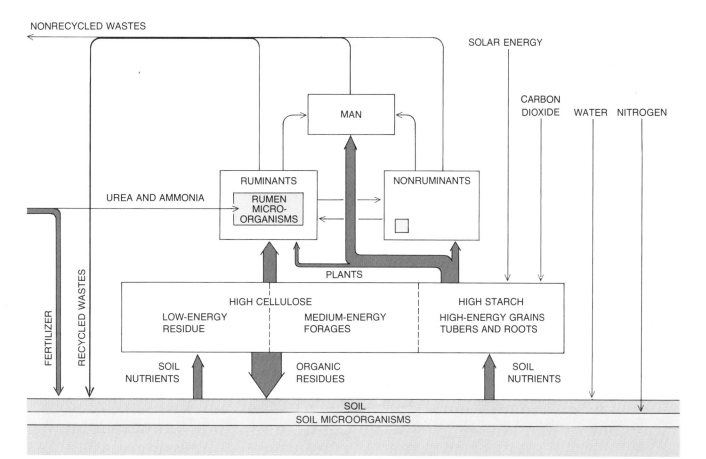

OVERALL NUTRIENT CYCLE includes man as the ultimate consumer and as the architect of the agricultural system. High-energy plant products, such as grains, are consumed by man directly or processed through animals. Lower-energy plant materials that are high in cellulose are processed through ruminants, thereby drawing on the capabilities of the rumen bacteria. The growth of the crops that support both the livestock and the human population is enhanced by returning wastes to the soil and by the application of fertilizers.

5

The Plants and Animals
That Nourish Man

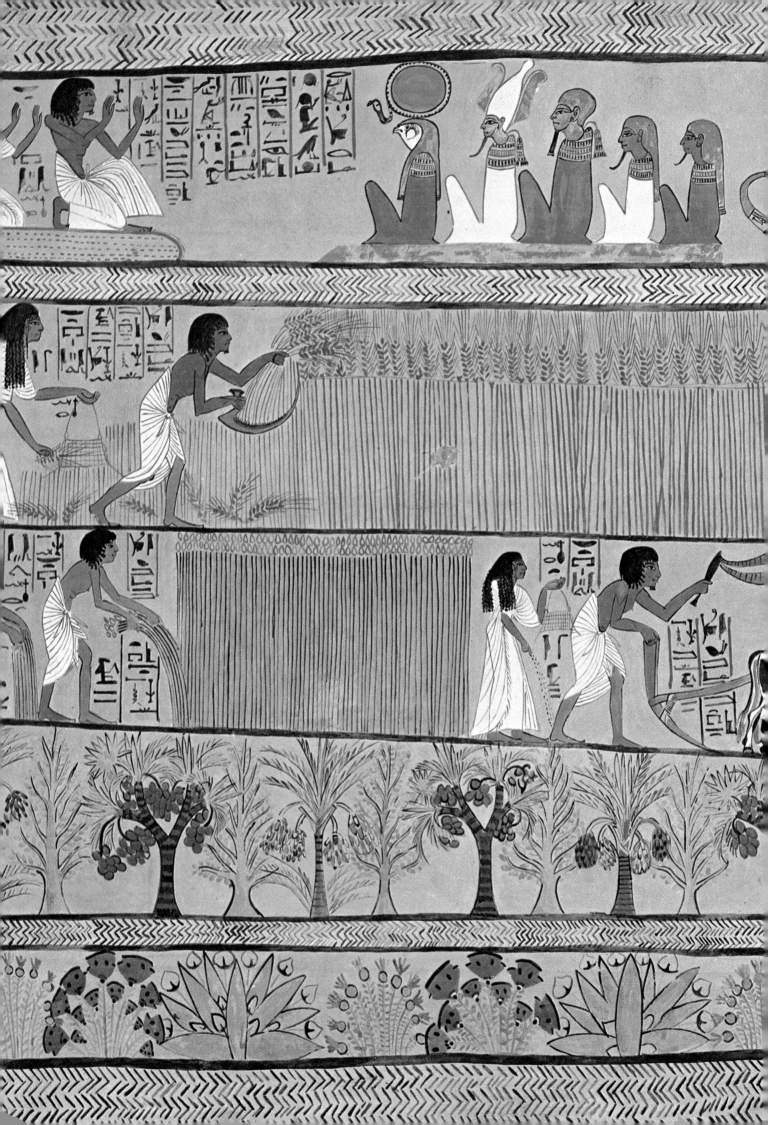

The Plants and Animals that Nourish Man

JACK R. HARLAN

Over the past 10,000 years man has chosen a relatively small number of plants and animals for domestication. The process made the domesticated species and man mutually dependent.

Man once enjoyed a highly varied diet. He has used for food several thousand species of plants and several hundred species of animals. Only a relatively small number of these species were ever domesticated. With the beginnings of agriculture there was a tendency to concentrate on the species that were the more productive and the most rewarding in terms of labor and capital invested. When towns and cities emerged, the list of food sources was narrowed somewhat as farmers sold the most profitable crops and animals to the urban population. In the past few centuries the trend has accelerated with industrialization and the rise of cash economies. The supermarket and quick-food services have drastically restricted the human diet in the U.S., and their influence is beginning to be felt abroad.

The trend for more and more people to be nourished by fewer and fewer plant and animal food sources has reached the point today where most of the world's population is absolutely dependent on a handful of species [*see illustration on next page*]. The four crops at the head of the list contribute more tonnage to the world total than the next 26 crops combined. This is a relatively recent phenomenon and was not characteristic of the traditional subsistence agricultures abandoned over the past few centuries. As the trend intensifies, man becomes ever more vulnerable. His food supply now depends on the success of a small number of species, and the failure of one of them may mean automatic starvation for millions of people. We have wandered down a path toward heavy dependence on a few species, and there seems to be no return.

Where, when and how did man begin this long and fateful journey? Twenty years ago the "where" was an easy question to answer. If one wanted to locate the origin of a domesticated plant, all one needed to do was to look it up in the writings of N. I. Vavilov, the geneticist who directed the All-Union Institute of Plant Industry in Leningrad from 1920 to 1940. Vavilov organized plant-collecting expeditions on a global scale, assembled masses of material, analyzed the collections and identified geographic "centers of origin" on the basis of the patterns of variation observed in both domestic crops and their wild relatives. He concluded that eight such centers existed, six of them in the Old World and two in the New.

Vavilov's work was monumental, and its impact on students of agriculture around the world was enormous. Studies since his time have shown, however, that the history of plant domestication is much more complicated than had been supposed. The weight of today's evidence is that many crops either did not originate in the centers Vavilov indicated or originated in more than one center. Some crops seem to have evolved over vast regions; there is no evidence at all

for a center of origin. Others cannot be pinned down with any precision for lack of suitable evidence.

In Vavilov's day scholars looked on agriculture as a revolutionary system of food procurement that had evolved on one or two hearths and diffused over the face of the earth, replacing the older hunting-gathering systems. The deliberate rearing of plants and animals for food was regarded as a discovery or invention so radical and so complex that it could have developed only once (or possibly twice), after which the system spread by stimulus diffusion. Hunting peoples coming into contact with farmers would instantly see and appreciate the enormous advantages of agriculture and hasten to go and do likewise. The evidence that has accumulated in recent years, particularly in the past decade, tends to suggest an almost opposite view. Agriculture is not an invention or a discovery and is not as revolutionary as we had thought; furthermore, it was adopted slowly and with reluctance.

The current evidence indicates that agriculture evolved through an extension and intensification of what people had already been doing for a long time. As we examine the domestication of plants and animals in more detail what once seemed to be well-defined centers tend to fade or to become vague and indistinct. My own viewpoint has changed with the evidence, and what I thought and wrote 20 years ago bears little resemblance to my present assessment of the situation.

The innovative pattern that now emerges is complex, diffuse and not easy to describe. For example, evidence for the domestication of pigs is found all the way from Europe to the Far East. Cattle of various kinds were tamed over most of the same range. With respect to plants, much the same is true of rice in Asia, of sorghum in Africa and of beans

CROPS OF EGYPT in the latter half of the second millennium B.C. appear in the painting on the opposite page; the original painting is in a tomb near the royal capital of Thebes. Areas with a herringbone pattern represent water. The tan grain being reaped with a sickle is an early species of wheat, emmer, the common wheat of Egypt until the fourth century B.C. The tall green crop in the panel below is flax; it is being uprooted, the usual harvesting method. To the right a plowman is cutting a furrow. A pair of oxen draw the plow, and the plowman's wife follows, dropping seed into the furrow. In the next panel the trees with clusters of small fruits are date palms and those with larger fruits are doum palms; the pale green trees between them are a species of fig, *Ficus sycomorus*, the sycamore of the Bible. Bottom panel shows water plants.

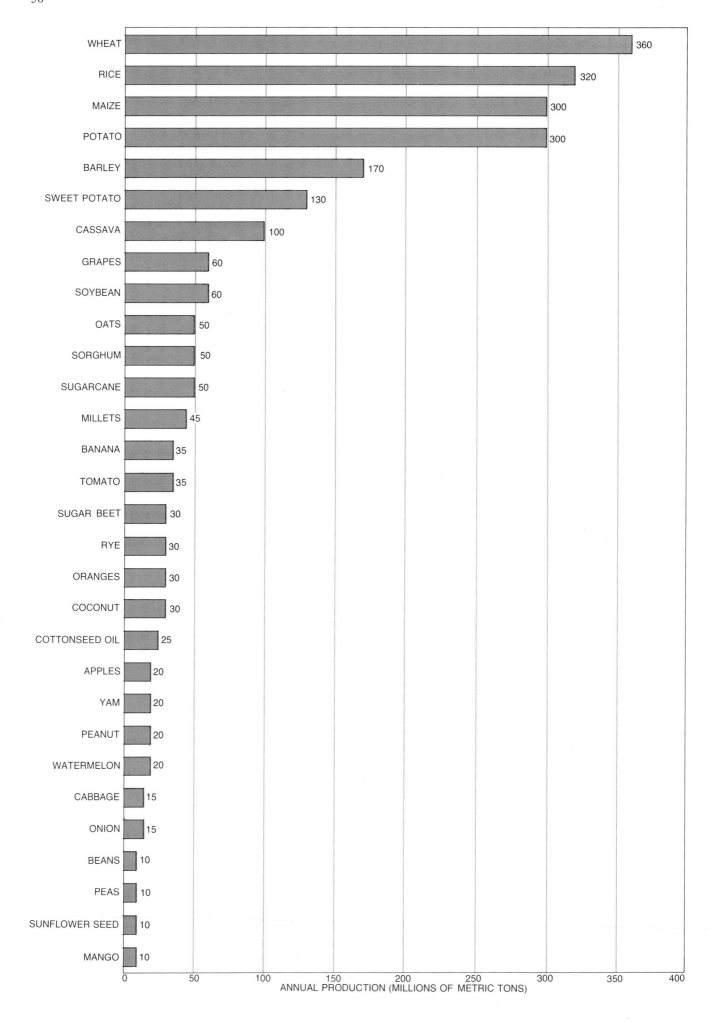

in the Americas [*see top illustration on next two pages*]. The wild progenitors of these food plants are widely distributed and were manipulated by various peoples over their entire range. Each may have been repeatedly domesticated at different times in different places or may have been brought into the domestic fold in several regions simultaneously. At least we cannot point with any confidence or precision to a single center of origin for these particular plants and animals.

By the same token, if the plant or animal under investigation never spread very far or did so only in recent historical times, the picture is usually rather clear and we can assign it an origin with some assurance. For example, two species of oxen, the mithan (*Bos gaurus*) and the yak (*Bos grunniens*), have rather modest ranges, and it seems likely they were domesticated within their present distribution: the mithan among the hill tribes of northwestern Burma, Assam and Bhutan, and the yak in Tibet and the adjacent highland regions. The sunflower was a rather minor crop grown by the Indians of what is now the U.S. It became a major oil crop in eastern Europe only recently. The African oil palm is another plant that has become important on the world scene only in the past few decades; its history is easily traced.

The possibility of independent domestications clearly complicates matters greatly. In some cases the evidence is nonetheless fairly clear. For example, it seems likely that the large-seed lima bean was domesticated in South America and the small-seed sieva bean in Mexico. One species of rice was domesticated in Asia and another in Africa. One species of cotton was domesticated in either India or Africa, another in South America and a third in Mesoamerica. Five species of squash and five of *Capsicum* peppers were domesticated over a geographic range that extends from Mexico to Argentina. Different species of yams were domesticated in West Africa, in Southeast Asia and in tropical America. Different races of radishes were independently domesticated in Japan, Indonesia, India and Europe. Where the species and races are clearly distinguishable we can usually unravel their history. Where we cannot clearly separate the races of a wild progenitor, however, the evidence for origins may be vague indeed. Moreover, in many instances the evidence is inadequate be-

THIRTY MAJOR CROPS include seven with annual harvests of 100 million or more metric tons. The total tonnage of the top seven crops is more than twice the tonnage of the remaining 23. Cane sugar and beet sugar are listed separately here but millets are combined. Crops with an annual yield of less than 10 million metric tons have been omitted.

cause we have failed to conduct serious investigations into the matter.

Such is probably the case for several crops with obscure origins. Old World cotton and the oilseed sesame could have either African or Indian origins or both. We do not know where, if anywhere, the bottle gourd genuinely grows wild. Indeed, it is often difficult to distinguish genuinely wild races from weedy escapes or naturalized races. In a few instances the original distribution patterns may have become so obscure that the evidence has disappeared.

Among the major food crops shown in the illustration on the opposite page several were of minor importance on the world scene until recently. The potato was restricted largely to the Andean highlands until the Europeans arrived there in the 16th century. It was brought to Europe soon afterward but was poorly adapted to local growing conditions and entered a period of acclimatization, particularly to the long-day regime characteristic of summers in Europe. Finally the potato found a congenial home and became so productive in northern Europe that it was credited by some historians with provoking something of a population explosion. From the world point of view such crops as sugarcane, the sugar beet, soybeans, citrus fruits, the tomato, the peanut, the sweet potato and the sunflower are all relatively recent major contributors to the food supply. Cottonseed as a major source of edible oil is a product of this century.

A point to be kept in mind when dealing with the "where" of domestication is that plants and animals under domestication change radically with time, and the forms familiar to us today may be strikingly different from the forms of the ancient progenitors. Wheat provides

a good example. Three kinds of wheat were originally domesticated from wild grasses; all three are so obsolete today that they are hardly grown at all. One was a diploid (that is, a plant with seven pairs of chromosomes) called einkorn. It was probably domesticated in southeastern Turkey, and it was always a minor crop. Einkorn did spread to western Europe, but it never reached Egypt, and it did not move eastward from its point of origin.

The second wheat was a tetraploid (that is, it had 14 pairs of chromosomes) called emmer. It was in its day by far the most successful of the three. Our best guess is that it originated in Palestine and/or southeastern Turkey. For some millenniums it was the dominant wheat. It spread across Europe and North Africa, Egypt and Arabia and reached Ethiopia, where it is still grown on a considerable scale. Emmer was the wheat of Egypt until it was replaced by bread wheat after Alexander the Great conquered Egypt in the fourth century B.C. Outside Ethiopia emmer lingers on as a relict crop in Yugoslavia and southern India.

The third domesticated wheat was also a tetraploid. It was so trivial that there is no common name for it; scientifically it is called *Triticum timopheevii*. It originated in Transcaucasian Georgia and has spread only as a collector's item for genetic studies.

The wheat we grow today is none of these three early domesticates. All three are known as glume wheats because the spike, or seed-bearing head, breaks up when it is threshed, leaving each seed enclosed in a hard, shell-like glume, or husk. The seeds must then be processed further, usually by pounding in a mortar, to free them of the husks. Some time after emmer was domesticated a mutation occurred that caused the base of the

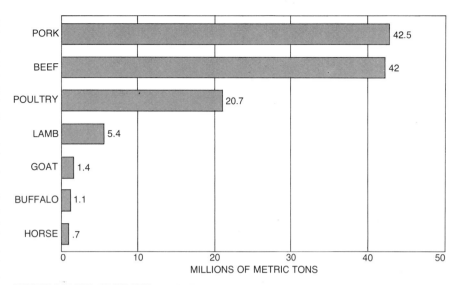

SEVEN MAJOR SOURCES provided a total of more than 110 million metric tons of meat worldwide in 1974, according to statistics from the Food and Agriculture Organization of the United Nations. The world pig population made the major contribution: 42.5 million tons. Beef and veal combined were in second place; chicken, duck and turkey combined were third.

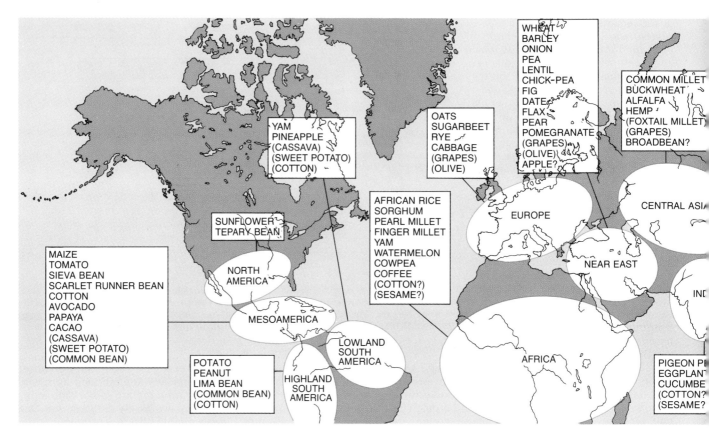

AREAS WHERE PLANTS WERE DOMESTICATED are indicated on this map; area boundaries have been generalized. Except for wheat, where different genera or species were independently domesticated in different areas, the name appears in each area; cotton, yams and the millets are examples. Where the same species was certainly or probably domesticated independently the name appears enclosed in parentheses in each area; among the examples are the common bean, the sweet potato, olive and grapes. Where the area of domesti-

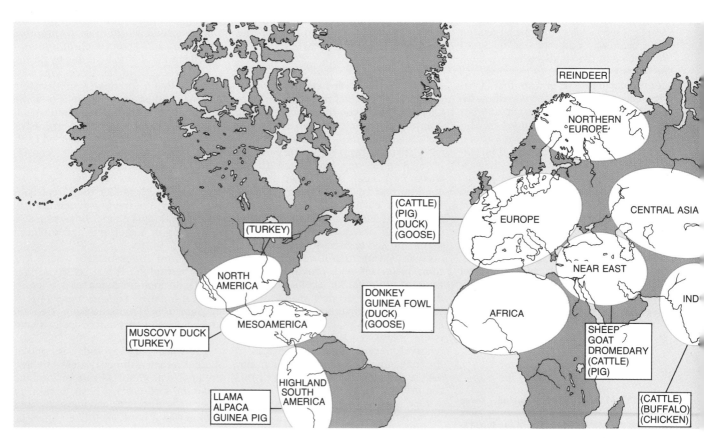

AREAS WHERE ANIMALS WERE DOMESTICATED are indicated on this map; as with the map showing plant domestication the area boundaries are generalized. In addition to the six species of mammals and the three species of birds that are man's most numerous domesticates, a number of animals valued for food, for work or for transport are also shown. The names of animals that were cer-

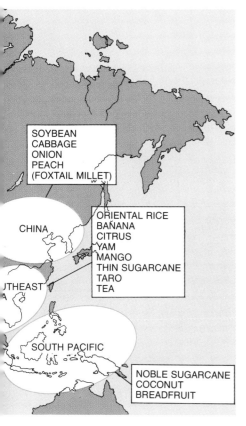

cation is in doubt a question mark follows the plant name. **Several crops with an annual yield below 10 million metric tons are included; examples are lentils, coffee and tea.**

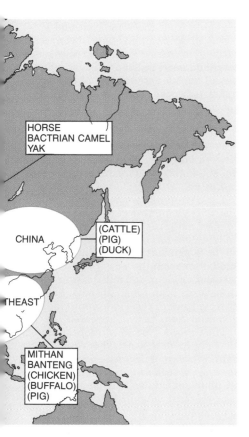

tainly or probably domesticated independently in more than one area are in parentheses: examples include pigs, cattle and chickens.

glume to collapse at maturity, freeing the seed. At the same time the spike became tough, so that it did not fall apart as the ancestral spikes had done. The mutated, free-threshing emmer is the ancestor of our durum or macaroni wheats.

The major wheat species of the world, and the one that contributes most to the annual harvest of 360 million metric tons, is still another kind, known generally as bread wheat. It is a hexaploid, that is, it has 21 pairs of chromosomes, and it arose long after the initial domestication of the three primitive glume wheats. Its extra set of chromosomes was contributed by a wild goat grass called *Triticum tauschii,* and the distribution of the wild progenitor suggests that the hybridization may have taken place somewhere near the southern end of the Caspian Sea. *T. tauschii* is the only species of goat grass with a continental distribution, and it may have contributed the adaptation that makes it possible for bread wheat to be grown on the dry steppes of the world. As a wild grass *T. tauschii* is essentially worthless, but as a contributor of genetic characteristics it literally made a billion-dollar crop out of a million-dollar one.

The word wheat, then, has several meanings. Modern wheats are quite different from the primitive glume wheats that were first domesticated. We can assign the origin of wheat to the Near East as long as we do not restrict the area too narrowly. The early evolution of wheat took place in a zone extending from Palestine to the Caucasus and the southern Caspian. Like all other domestic plants, however, wheat is still evolving and changing wherever it grows today.

It is now possible to list in similar fashion other major domesticated plants and animals, along with our best guess as to their geographic origins. In a number of cases, however, it is necessary to include the same species in more than one region because of diffuse patterns of domestication, and in some instances we must resort to question marks because of ignorance.

We are not much better off with our answers to the "when" of domestication, although each year brings some new knowledge. For example, it has often been said that the dog was the first animal to be domesticated. Until recently we had no firm evidence for this belief, but the jaws and teeth of domestic dogs have now been identified and dated to about 12,000 B.C. in the Old World (Iraq) and to about 11,000 B.C. in the New World (Idaho). Dogs have been eaten by man on every continent, but they were probably never considered a major meat animal except in parts of the New World before the arrival of the Europeans.

Apart from the two dog dates we see

little evidence for animal domestication until about 9000 B.C. Even here the data are rather tenuous and not conclusive. Zawi Chemi Shanidar is an archaeological site in Iraq that was excavated by Ralph S. Solecki in the 1960's; the animal bones unearthed there were analyzed by Dexter Perkins, Jr. Now, if one finds the right bones, it is possible to distinguish between sheep and goats that are less than a year old and those that are more than a year old. Near the bottom of Solecki's excavations the remains of both sheep and goats less than a year old made up about 25 percent of the sample. Toward the top, where the remains were more recent, there was a shift to a higher ratio of sheep bones to goat bones, and about 50 percent of the sheep were less than a year old. The implication is that the people at Shanidar had acquired considerable control over the sheep population but not over the goat population.

It is also possible, given the right bones, to determine the sex of an animal. At some archaeological sites it has been found that the bones of a high percentage of young male animals are present. This does not in itself prove domestication; similarly displaced sex and age ratios are found among the remains of red deer in European Mesolithic sites and the remains of gazelles at Near Eastern sites. Both are considered game animals, but both can be tamed. Evidence for domestication is difficult to obtain from bones unless changes in morphology are involved. Such findings do, however, suggest manipulation of some kind, and they certainly indicate that as far back as the Mesolithic man had both the capacity and the technique for selective slaughtering. This in turn was probably a first step in an increasingly intimate interaction of man with his food animals.

A second Near Eastern archaeological site, Ali Kosh in Iran, may have been occupied as early as 7500 B.C. The dating of its lower levels is uncertain, but the skull of a hornless female sheep was unearthed in one of the lowest. In wild sheep both sexes have horns, so that the hornless skull is taken to mean that domestic sheep were present at Ali Kosh. Goat bones are much more abundant at the site than sheep bones, and a high percentage represent young males.

Çayönü, an early farming village in Turkey, was first excavated by Robert J. Braidwood and Halet Çambel in 1964. It was first inhabited perhaps a little before 7000 B.C.; the bones of domestic sheep, pigs, dogs and probably goats were present. Remains of domestic goats with twisted horns are present at the site of Jarmo in Iraq, a site dating to about 6750 B.C. Twisted horns are characteristic of domesticated breeds and not of wild goats.

The earliest remains of domesticated

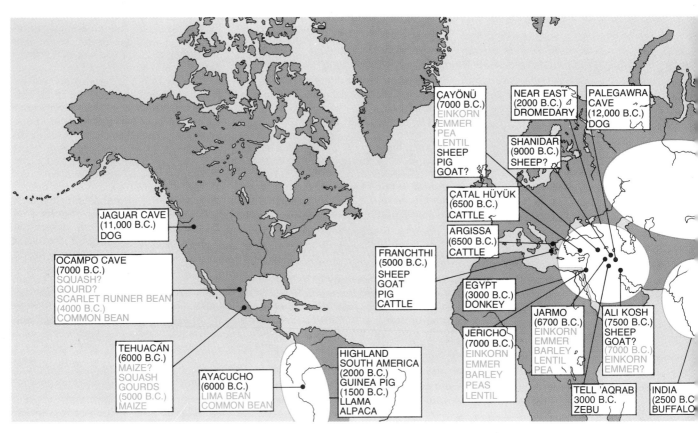

EARLIEST DOMESTICATIONS of plants and animals appear to have taken place at roughly the same time around the world. Shown on the map are general Old World and New World areas or specific archaeological sites where the remains of plants (*color*) and animals

cattle now known come from Greece and date to about 6500 B.C. By then this species of animal apparently had long been worshiped. At Çatal Hüyük, a Turkish site excavated by James Mellaart and dated about 6500 B.C., more than 50 shrines were uncovered; most of them were decorated with bull's heads and horns. The humped cattle we associate with India today are represented by Mesopotamian figurines dating back to about 3000 B.C.; they are not recorded in India until about 2500 B.C. We have no information on the antiquity of other bovids, such as the banteng (*Bos javanicus*) of Malaysia, the mithan and the yak. The water buffalo was known as a domesticate in India by 2500 B.C., but it could have been a source of draft power, meat and milk long before then.

The donkey was known as a domesticate in Egypt by 3000 B.C. and may have been exploited well before that; it has not been used much as a food animal. The horse, in contrast, has been an important source of meat and milk for many peoples. Fermented mare's milk is still popular in Asia, and half a million metric tons of horsemeat are eaten worldwide each year [*see illustration on page 59*]. The horse is thought to have first been tamed in central Asia or southern Russia about 3000 B.C. The reindeer, a domesticate now commonest in Scandinavia and the U.S.S.R., was probably herded at a very early date, but we have

no firm evidence for it. Among the camelids our best guesses suggest 2000 B.C. for the one-humped dromedary and 1500 B.C. for the two-humped Bactrian camel; about the same time range probably applies to the New World camelids, the llama and the alpaca. The guinea pig of the Andes was probably a tamed food animal by 2000 B.C.

Many Near Eastern sites have also yielded early plant remains. None appear at Shanidar, but Ali Kosh yielded grains of einkorn and emmer wheats that date back to about 7000 B.C. and barley that is somewhat younger. Seeds of einkorn, emmer, pea, lentil, vetch and flax were found at Çayönü. Jarmo had einkorn, emmer, barley, pea, lentil and vetch, and a similar array of plant foods was found in the prepottery Neolithic levels at Jericho, which are also dated at about 7000 B.C. Other sites document rather clearly a progression of farming into Greece and the Balkans and thereafter a fanning out over Europe.

The bias in our data has led many to conclude that the Near East was the center of Old World plant and animal domestication. We have a fairly respectable body of information for that part of the world and an even better record for Europe. Some caution is advisable, however; no other parts of the world have been as well explored (except North America, where agriculture ar-

rived comparatively late). For example, we have almost no archaeological information from Africa of the kind that is available from the Near East and Europe. Plant remains have been unearthed in Africa, including those of sorghum, pearl millet and finger millet, but all the sites are too recent to tell us much. Indirect evidence, such as the discovery of mortars and grinding stones and of flint blades with a particular kind of sheen or gloss, which might have been used to reap grasses, appears in the Nile Valley by about 12,000 B.C., but we do not know what plants were being processed.

The situation is much the same in India, where a number of sites have yielded plant materials but where most of the finds are too recent to yield information on the beginnings of agriculture. Wheat and barley from the west, rice from the east and sorghum and millets from Africa have all been found in India, but no firm evidence of early indigenous Indian domestications has yet appeared.

The Chinese Neolithic has been studied on a modest scale. The Yang Shao culture is now fairly well known, and some sites, such as Pan P'o, have yielded plant materials. This Neolithic village was first inhabited, however, only around 4000 B.C. Moreover, it contains some rather elegant pottery and appears much too large, complex and sophisticated to represent the beginnings of ag-

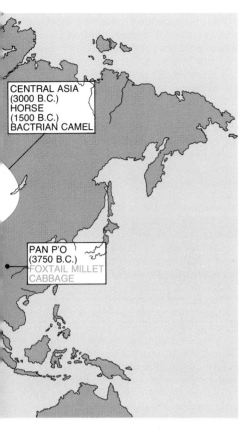

CENTRAL ASIA
(3000 B.C.)
HORSE
(1500 B.C.)
BACTRIAN CAMEL

PAN P'O
(3750 B.C.)
FOXTAIL MILLET
CABBAGE

suggest or confirm domestication at the date indicated. Data imply independent invention.

riculture in the Far East. Foxtail millet was the chief food crop of that time and place.

Work in Southeast Asia has for all practical purposes just begun. Early plant materials have been found at sites in Thailand, and there is even evidence for early landform manipulation in remote New Guinea. At present the body of information is too meager and fragmentary to allow the drawing of definite conclusions. Nevertheless, there are hints that the inhabitants of the region were manipulating plants quite as early as the people of the Near East.

The situation in the Americas is not much better and not much different. Enormous quantities of beautifully preserved plant materials are available from coastal Peru, but this is not a likely region for agricultural innovation. Excavations in Tamaulipas and in the Tehuacán valley in Mexico by Richard S. MacNeish have given us sequences of deposits suggesting plant manipulation about 7000 B.C., and some later material on domesticates, possibly dating back to 6000 B.C. and surely to 5000 B.C. Maize was apparently a crop in Tehuacán by then, along with squash and gourds, and beans appeared before 3000 B.C. Tehuacán is too dry, however, to have been a center of agricultural developments. It seems more likely that events taking place elsewhere were sometimes recorded there and that the valley itself was

outside the mainstream of agricultural innovation. MacNeish's investigations at Ayacucho in Peru are perhaps more revealing. Although he failed to find evidence of early agriculture in the Andean highlands, he did find plant materials in the intermontane valleys. By 6000 B.C. fully domesticated beans and lima beans were being cultivated there. Thus agriculture could well be as ancient a tradition in South America as it is in the Near East and in Southeast Asia, although conclusive evidence of it is not available at present.

On balance, then, the evidence for "when," such as it is, seems to be as diffuse and imprecise as the evidence for "where." This is only partly owing to inadequate investigation. Some of the uncertainties are surely the result of the way domestication took place. For reasons we can only speculate about, people in various parts of the world all seem to have begun the processes of domestication at roughly the same time. That time was not long after the final Pleistocene glaciation, when the great ice sheets had melted and the seas had risen to approximately their present levels. It would not be appropriate to pursue the various speculations here; it is enough to say that the picture now emerging in terms of both time and place turns out to be far more complex and diffuse than we used to think.

With both the where and the when of domestication left somewhat up in the air, what is there to say about how? One can begin by pointing out that plant cultivation and plant domestication are often confused. Cultivation refers to man's efforts to care for plants; in this sense it is perfectly possible to cultivate wild plants. Domestication, from *domus,* the Latin for house, means to bring into the household, and hence it implies far more than cultivation. Domestication involves genetic changes that make the plants better suited to the conditions of man-made environments and less well adapted to the conditions of natural environments. In a similar way one can tame a wild animal without domesticating it. The genetic alteration that is involved in the process of domestication, however, is often carried to the point where a fully domesticated plant or animal is fitted exclusively to an artificial environment and cannot survive in the wild.

Horses, cattle and camels have escaped from domestication in western North America in historic times and have thrived. Sheep that escape from domestication, on the other hand, have little chance of survival unless they are protected from predators. Goats that escape thrive in the absence of predators, as when they escape to an island; when predators are present, they fare poor-

ly. Similarly, the domesticated races of maize, wheat, rice, potato, sweet potato and most other crops would all die out without human intervention.

Because domestication is an evolutionary process it is variable in degree, and one finds an entire range of intermediate states from wild races to fully domesticated races that depend entirely on man for survival. Indeed, all these intermediate states may be found in the same species. There are wild, weedy and domesticated races of most of our crops. The wild ones can survive without man, the weedy races survive because of man (and in spite of his efforts to get rid of them) and the domesticated races demand care and cultivation for survival. Weeds are species or races that thrive in man-made habitats; most of our crops have weed races somewhere. There are weed races of wheat, rice, maize, potato, barley and so on, all the way down the list. They readily propagate themselves, but they require habitats that are disturbed by man.

This kind of adaptation is not confined to plants. Cats, dogs and pigs readily become feral. The statuary pigeon, the house sparrow and the starling thrive even in the face of intense human disturbance, as they do in cities. The house mouse, the sewer rat, the housefly and the fruit fly all do well in the artificial habitats created by man. Indeed, what species thrives in man-made habitats better than *Homo sapiens?* We are the weediest of all.

Recent studies of weed races show that their origins may be diverse. Even genuinely wild plants can show weedy tendencies; after all, many natural environments such as shorelines, riverbanks, the margins of glaciers and steep talus slopes are unstable, whereas others are subject to disturbances such as forest fires, blowdowns, avalanches and the like. Many wild species occupy these niches, and some of our crop plants are derived from wild plants with just such colonizer tendencies. Other weeds are derived from natural crosses between wild and domesticated races and still others come from the escape of half-domesticated plants. Hybridization between cultivated plants and related weed races has played a role in crop evolution by increasing diversity and developing efficient population structures. Similar genetic interactions of domestic animals and their wild relatives were probably an important element in the early days of animal husbandry. The process is now relatively uncommon because the related wild races have become rare or extinct, but in Southeast Asia chickens still mate with jungle fowl and in New Guinea tame sows are frequently serviced by wild boars.

The process of plant domestication presumably began with man's intensive use of and at least partial dependence on the plant in question. The relationship inevitably increased in intimacy. For example, man's harvesting of seeds from wild plants would have had relatively little effect on the genetic structure of the wild plant populations until man himself sowed what he had reaped. Once seed is deliberately planted the composition of the next plant generation depends on what man harvests, and so some genetic changes become virtually automatic. The most common genetic response in crops valued for their edible seed is a shift toward nonshattering, that is, a shift away from natural seed dispersal. Cereal panicles and spikes become tough and do not break apart at maturity. Pods and capsules no longer burst open to disperse their seeds when they are ripe. Once the natural mechanism for seed dispersal is lost the plants become dependent on man for survival. They are domesticated, or at least partly so. The genetic change may be very simple and is frequently controlled by a single gene.

Other changes also take place more or less automatically. The seeds of wild plants are often dormant at maturity, and even if conditions are favorable for germination, they will not germinate until the proper season. This is an elegant adaptation for wild species, but it may not be at all suitable for agriculture. When this is the case, selection for nondormancy, or at least for a dormancy that breaks down by the next planting time, is automatic. By the same token automatic selection for larger seeds will occur in the seedbeds if there is competition between seedlings. Large seeds have larger food reserves and are likely to produce more vigorous seedlings; the first plants to come up and those with the greatest seedling vigor are likely to contribute the most seed to the next generation. Still other automatic selection pressures adapt plants to field conditions. A disruptive selection is set up: natural selection causes the wild populations to maintain their adaptations, but repeated sowing and reaping modify the cultivated populations in the direction of adaptation to field and garden. Genetic divergence is easily maintained even when there is considerable crossing between the wild and the cultivated populations.

In addition to the automatic selection pressures, man intervenes by deliberate and intentional processes of selection. These processes may aim in different directions and may be capricious, to say the least. Man selects corn for boiling, for popping, for roasting in the ear, for flour quality, for making hominy, for beer, for unfermented beverages, for dyes and even for ceremonial and religious purposes. He selects nonglutinous and glutinous rice, long-grained and short-grained rice, red rice, white rice and aromatic rice. He selects barley for food, for beer, for livestock feed, for processing in his grinding equipment and for ease of harvesting. Man delights in bright colors and in curious and unusual variants, and so he preserves plant forms that would have no chance of survival under natural conditions.

The part of the plant of greatest interest to man is the part that is modified the most. If the crop is a tuber, the greatest variation and the greatest deviation from the wild type will be in the tuber. If it is a cereal, the parts most modified will be the inflorescence and the grains borne on it. A striking example is the kale species, *Brassica oleracea*, which as a result of man's influence has been modified in half a dozen ways. The species has a remarkable capacity for developing starch-storage organs on demand. In the familiar cabbage the storage organ is the terminal bud; in the cauliflower it is the inflorescence, in kohlrabi the stem, in Brussels sprouts the lateral buds, in broccoli the stems and flowers and in kale the leaves. All evolved by selection from the wild *B. oleracea*. Different as these plants are in appearance, they are all the same species and are fully fertile when they are hybridized. Kale is closer to the wild type than the others.

Beets provide another example: the garden beet, the mangel or fodder beet, the sugar beet and the leafy green Swiss chard are all derivative forms of *Beta vulgaris*. Some peoples selected for the leaves, some for the roots and some for the sugar. Still other examples are legion. The variation in lettuces in a neighborhood market in Italy is surprising to those of us who see only the lettuces offered in an American supermarket. Selection strategies in beans have taken two major forms: dry beans and green beans. The strategies in peas include not only dry and green forms but also pod (or snow) peas. The end result of such intense and divergent selection pressures is the production of morphological monsters that are completely dependent on man for survival; these plants are fully domesticated.

The domestication of animals is no different in principle. The process begins with an intimate relation between man and an animal and a partial dependence of man on the animal. This may involve a selective kind of hunting or the

SPECIES OF WHEAT include, from left to right, the three earliest domesticates: einkorn (*Triticum monococcum*), once grown in Turkey and Europe, emmer (*T. dicoccum*), once grown in the Near East, Africa and Europe, and a third with no common name, *T. timopheevii*. Next are the principal modern wheats: macaroni wheat (*T. durum*), a descendant of a mutated emmer, and bread wheat (*T. aestivum*), a cross between emmer or macaroni wheat and goat grass.

management of a herd. Sooner or later the animals are tamed. It is usually not difficult. Young animals that are raised in or near the household often become tame for life. Some animal species are recalcitrant and difficult to tame, but many that have never been domesticated prove to be quite tractable. In the course of domestication there has doubtless been some selection for genes conferring docility. In cattle and pigs selection led to smaller animals that were easier to handle, and dwarf breeds of several other domestic animals have also been developed.

Recent experience may serve as a model of what probably happened in the deep past. For example, the musk-ox has been tamed to allow access to its extraordinarily fine wool. The project was designed to provide income for Eskimos and other northern populations whose traditional hunting cultures had been disrupted. In spite of a reputation for belligerency the musk-ox has proved to be tractable and docile under artificial husbandry. As another example, about a century ago the African eland was introduced into Russia on a trial basis. It adapted to confinement very well, and selection for milk production resulted in a more than 400 percent increase over the production of animals in the wild state. The milking eland could be called a modern domesticate.

Selective breeding of tamed or confined animals leads eventually to domesticated races and lineages that cannot survive in nature even if the species itself could manage without the aid of man. Extreme types such as the Pekingese dog, the bubble-eyed goldfish, chickens with five-meter feathers, pouter pigeons, waltzing mice and for that matter most strains of laboratory mice, rats, rabbits and mutant stocks of fruit flies have been genetically modified to the point where they depend on man for survival and are fully domesticated.

If total dependence is a consequence of domestication, what is one to say of the human condition? Man likes to think that he is in charge of the plants and animals he first began to bring into his household several thousand years ago, but the fact is that he has been domesticated by them. Many of them cannot now survive without man, but certainly they are essential to man's survival. More precisely, man and his domesticates have been bound together for some millenniums in an adaptive coevolution. Human evolution, in its peculiar way, is largely social and cultural, whereas the evolution of man's plant and animal domesticates has involved notable genetic changes and the development of striking new morphologies. Although man must care for his domesticates, the human population of the world eats or starves according to the performance of those few plants and animals that nourish man.

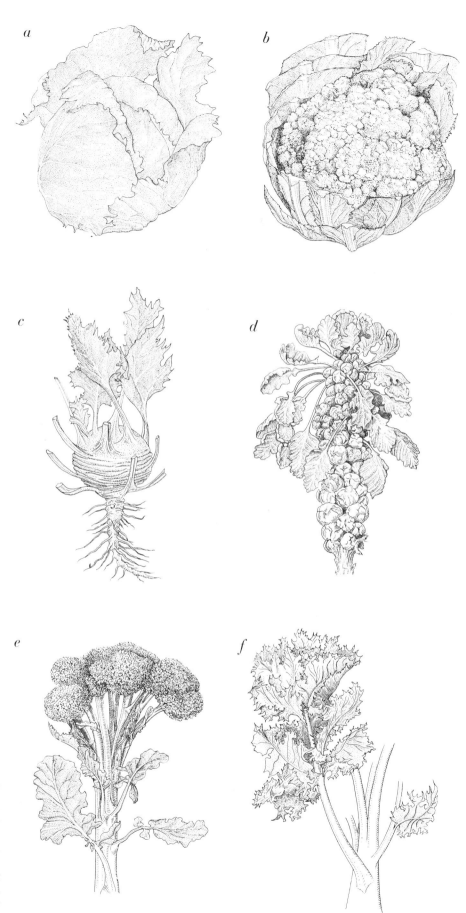

PRESSURE OF SELECTION has produced six separate vegetables from a single species, *Brassica oleracea*, a mustard with a remarkable capacity for developing starch-storage organs on demand. Selection for enlarged terminal buds produced the cabbage (*a*); for inflorescences, the cauliflower (*b*); for the stem, kohlrabi (*c*); for lateral buds, Brussels sprouts (*d*); for the stem and flowers, broccoli (*e*), and for leaves, kale (*f*). Kale most closely resembles the wild plant.

6

Agricultural Systems

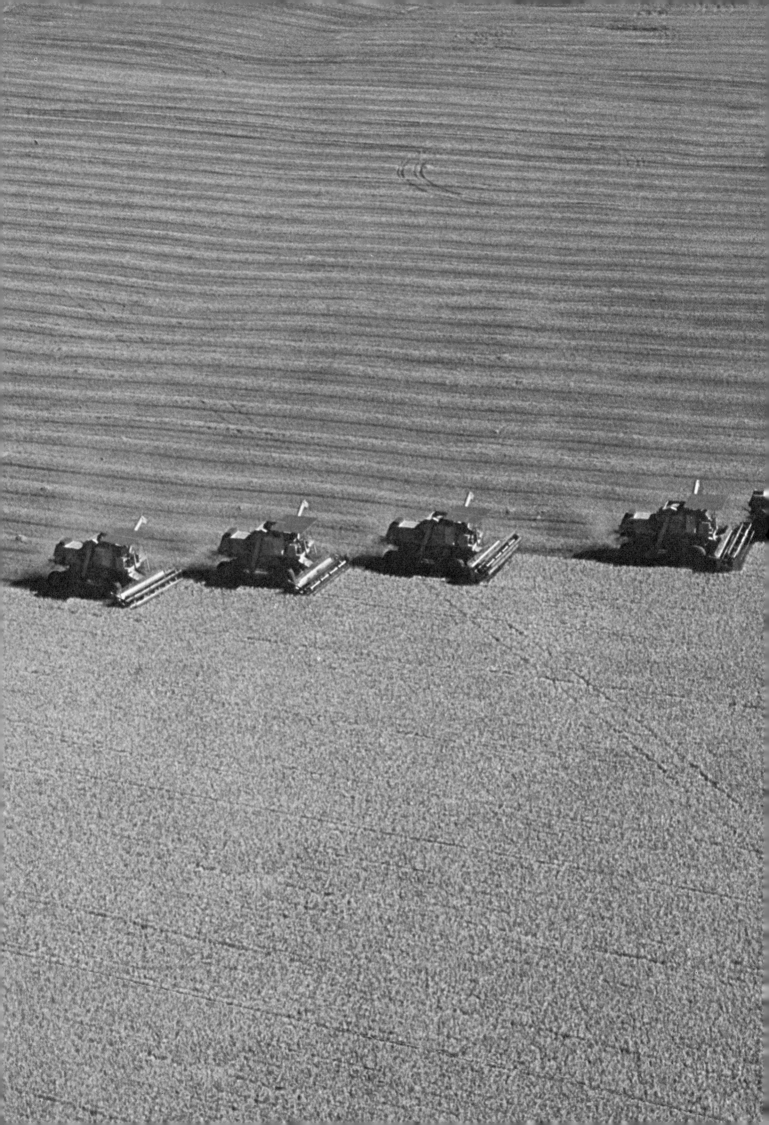

Agricultural Systems

They are established by a combination of ecological, economic and cultural factors. The problem today is how the developing countries can promote high-yielding systems based on cereals

In the U.S. one speaks of the corn belt and the wheat belt, reflecting the role of those plants as the principal crop in certain areas. Agricultural systems in other parts of the world can be similarly characterized by their dominant crops. In every such area, however, other crops are grown too, sometimes in rather intricate associations with the main crop. The agricultural pattern that has emerged in each area is in part the result of ecological factors—a particular combination of climate and soil—and in part the result of economic and cultural factors in the society that grows the crops.

Within each broad region one finds a considerable variation in farming practice. The farms vary in size, in intensity of management and in the types of secondary crop and livestock associated with the dominant crop. Notwithstanding the diversity in farming systems, there really are only four basic approaches to cropping. They can be characterized by the type of cultivation involved. The first approach is concerned with perennial tree or vine crops and is represented by such agricultural enterprises as orchards, vineyards and rubber plantations. In the second approach the emphasis is on cultivated crops such as corn and wheat, which are replanted in freshly tilled soil after harvest. The third approach is the grazing of permanent grassland, and the fourth entails the alternation of cultivated crops with grass or some other forage crop.

A close look at three cropping systems reveals some of the ecological factors that influence patterns of agriculture. The North American corn belt is a region devoted principally to cultivated crops, with corn (grown for its grain) the most important product. The region has large expanses in which the land is level

and the soil is fertile and well drained. They are mostly sown to corn, with soybeans an important second crop. In hilly areas that have poor soil and are subject to erosion the tendency is to rotate the major crops with sod-forming forage crops such as alfalfa. The poorest sites are left in permanent pasture of "native" bluegrass or seeded with superior grasses and legumes for intensive grazing.

Climate has a great deal to do with the emphasis on corn. A warm season with at least 120 days when the temperature is above 10 degrees Celsius (50 degrees Fahrenheit) is required, together with ample moisture well distributed over the season. Central Iowa and Illinois meet these requirements well. In central Minnesota the crop is limited by low temperatures, whereas in eastern Nebraska the limiting factor is scanty rainfall. The importance of corn in the eastern and southern regions of the U.S. has been limited in part by lower soil fertility. Corn is a major crop in several other parts of the world: Mexico, the Central American countries, Argentina, Indonesia, Thailand and parts of Europe, particularly the Balkan states.

On the Western plains of the U.S. the supply of moisture is inadequate for corn, which is therefore grown only where irrigation is possible. The wheat plant, which dominates the semiarid croplands of the world, fills the need in this area for a cultivated crop with a lower demand for water and a greater tolerance of drought. In the semiarid regions of Africa and also in parts of India and the U.S. Southwest, where the limited amount of rain falls mostly during the warm season, sorghum and millet are common as drought-tolerant grain crops.

Wheat, unlike corn and millet, grows

well during the cool weather of spring and fall, when evaporation is low and the plant's demand for moisture is therefore moderate. On the southern plains (Oklahoma and Kansas) the common practice is to plant "winter" wheat in the fall. The crop flowers and produces grain in the spring after being vernalized, or induced to flower, by the low temperatures in winter. Farther north, where wheat fails to survive the severer winters, spring wheat, which does not require vernalization, is planted early in the spring.

Varieties of wheat that mature early can be extended into environments where the rainfall is quite low. In the driest regions wheat is cropped only in alternate years. Between crops the land is left fallow and kept free of vegetation for a year so that the moisture of the soil can be restored to a level that will support the next wheat crop. As in corn systems, marginal lands are given over to grazing. The land's productivity of grass is low, so that the grazing activity on a Western cattle ranch involves a low density of animals.

The intensive grazing systems of the Netherlands and Denmark offer a distinct contrast to the cultivated-crop systems that yield corn and wheat. Low-lying, heavy soils in the region are usually too cold and wet for cultivated crops. They are therefore seeded to perennial ryegrass, a shallow-rooted species that grows well in cool weather and gives good production from the middle of spring to the middle of fall.

The farm practice in the region includes heavy fertilization and carefully controlled rotational grazing. Animals are turned into several pastures in sequence, so that each pasture has a period of time to recover after being grazed intensively. Part of the grassland is commonly harvested for hay or silage, which supplies feed during the winter. In other parts of the world a legume is frequently included in the pasture as a source of nitrogen. The species of grass and legumes are chosen for their adap-

CROP OF WHEAT is harvested by a group of combines in the eastern uplands of the state of Washington. The harvest scene is typical of the large-scale operations that also prevail in the wheat belts of the North American Great Plains, the U.S.S.R. and a number of other regions.

tation to the local climate and soil conditions.

With these three systems one sees that several factors act together to put ecological constraints on what can be grown in a particular area. They include the level and seasonal distribution of sunlight, temperature and rain, the condition of the soil, the topography of the land and the types of pest and disease to which the crop will be exposed. These factors determine whether it is feasible to introduce a certain crop in a given area. The actual choice of crops, however, is heavily dependent on the economic and cultural environment of the society that is doing the farming. So are the manner and intensity of cultivation. What one finds is that the density of the population, the distance to the market, the level of technology and the society's cultural heritage seem to play as large a role as natural forces.

Social factors cannot be completely separated in an analysis of farming systems for the simple reason that agriculture and the rest of the social system evolved together. Strong feedback interactions bring about a continual "tuning" of each sector. The present farming systems are the survivors of an enormous amount of human experimentation. Over the millenniums man has eaten the produce of several thousands of plants, several hundred of which have been domesticated. The emphasis in farming has been on plants that give a high return of storable product per unit of human effort, that are "safe" because their biological performance is reasonably consistent and that satisfy basic nutritional needs.

Our concern now is for the adequacy of these systems in the future. We need to know whether they have sufficient flexibility, safety and potential yield for rapidly expanding populations. The answers to these questions can be sought in an examination of agriculture as a system of food chains leading up to man, of how certain crops came to dominate particular farming systems and of how plant nutrition and social factors may be the most important considerations for the future of mankind.

Man as a flexible omnivore can place himself anywhere along a chain of animals subsisting on vegetation. The actual chain is usually rather short, involving either the direct consumption of vegetation or the eating of animal products from other primary consumers. Livestock play key roles in many farming systems; indeed, the principal complexity of agriculture has to do with the type of animal raised and with the relative emphasis given to food crops and feed crops. The channeling of organic production is aided by controlling the number of competing plants (weeds) and animals (such as insects) and by emphasizing a high efficiency of transfer of the natural resources and photosynthetic productivity that go into food production.

The simplest food chain is to grow plants and eat them (or parts of them). The efficiency of transfer of energy and protein can be very high in such a chain, with the result that a dense human population can be supported. It is common to find that from 30 to 40 percent of the net production of plants can be harvested as food and that from 70 to 80 percent of the harvest can be digested by man. Many of the numbers are smaller, however, so that there is considerable room for improvement. The most should be made of a plant's photosynthetic productivity while making sure that as much as possible of it goes into edible yield rather than into maintenance activity and residues.

An analogous problem in partitioning arises with the chemical composition of food materials. The protein content of various plant foods varies from about 6 percent to more than 20 percent of the dry matter. Systems based on a relatively low yield of protein have a distinct advantage, since a greater total yield of food is obtained per unit of area (that is, per unit of sunlight, water or soil nitrogen) or per unit of effort. The production of protein by a plant involves energy-expensive biochemical steps such as the uptake and reduction of nitrate nitrogen. The energy comes from carbohydrates that otherwise would accumulate as food. As a result the total organic yield of a crop is often inversely related to its protein content. Low-protein plant materials can be quite satisfactory as food. A diet of cereal grains with only from 10 to 12 percent protein (by weight) is nutritionally adequate for adults in protein and essential amino acids. Indeed, human diets are at present more limited by their content of energy (calories) than by their content of protein.

The evolution of agriculture based on cereals fits this concept. Small grains (wheat, barley, rye, oats and rice) and large grains (corn, sorghum and some millets) collectively provide directly more than 50 percent of the world's pro-

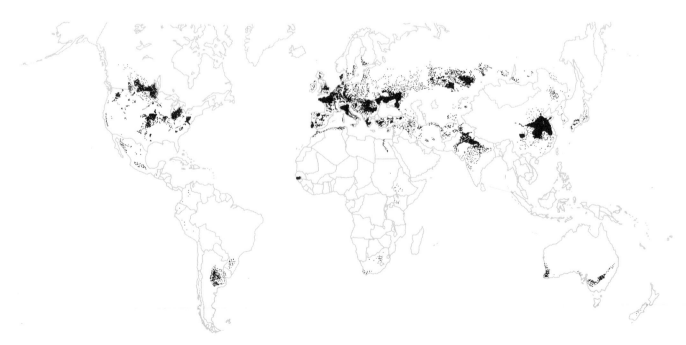

MAJOR WHEAT ZONES of the world are shown in black. Each dot represents 27,000 metric tons; the total in the world is about 350 million metric tons per year (13 billion bushels). This map and the next two are based on data from the U.S. Department of Agriculture.

tein and energy needs. Taking into account the large amounts of grain that are converted by livestock into meat, milk and eggs and by microorganisms into alcoholic beverages and other products, one finds that 75 percent of the energy and protein needs of man are met by cultivated grains.

The heavy emphasis on cereals reflects not only their food value but also their relative ease of culture, harvest, transport and storage, and their wide range of climatic adaptation. Moreover, cereals are fairly plastic in their response to climate, and they mature within a relatively short growing season, so that their vulnerability to unseasonal weather is low.

In the Tropics, where storage is difficult and the growing season is long, farming systems tend to emphasize everbearing plants and year-round sequences of food crops. Root and tuber crops such as potatoes, manioc, yams and taro suit these systems. They provide about 8 percent of the energy and 5 percent of the protein that man derives from food. Peas, beans, nuts and oilseeds contribute 5 percent of the energy and 12 percent of the protein, and sugar crops contribute about 9 percent of the energy. According to data compiled by the Food and Agriculture Organization of the United Nations, other fruits and vegetables account for only 2 percent of caloric needs and less than 1 percent of the protein requirement. The figures probably underestimate the importance of these foods in the Tropics, and the numbers would rise if the produce of domestic gardens were counted in the statistics. The minor ranking of these crops is related in part to the prob-

lems of transporting and storing fresh produce.

On a worldwide basis the human species now relies on 11 plant species for about 80 percent of its food supply. This base is not as limited as it might seem. Most of the plant species represent enormous genetic complexes; some, such as wheat and corn, have more diversity than is found in all but a few wild species. Retaining and extending this diversity are important matters to agricultural scientists, among whom it is widely agreed that efforts in this direction should be increased considerably.

Moreover, most of the species on which man relies are capable of flourishing in a variety of environments, so that a considerable amount of substitution in culture and use is possible. For example, although wheat is gradually displacing rye, barley and oats from their traditional role as Temperate Zone food crops, they remain (along with corn and potatoes) alternatives for the region. Triticale, a new species arising from hybrids of wheat and rye, also has the appropriate traits. In the event of a failure of a crop such as wheat the solution lies more with man's perception of the event, his willingness to change and his speed in making the change than it does with the issue of whether or not enough alternatives exist.

The dominance of a certain crop in a certain region comes about as a result of the integration of a number of economic and ecological factors. The dominant crop is well adapted to the environment and gives a high yield. It also fits well into a plan of farm management and has a relatively low risk of failure. A

market is available that makes it possible for the crop to serve as the basis for a good income to the farmer. In short, the system has been tuned to local conditions.

The incentives to extend a successful cropping system into marginal environments are strong. In the fringe areas, where the crop's vulnerability to weather is higher and its yields are lower, it may be replaced as the main crop by another system centered on a safer crop. Forces of this kind are involved in the replacement of corn by wheat in areas with low rainfall. One result of the tendency to move into fringe areas is that agricultural research in the U.S. has been much concerned with developing plants that will be able to withstand the relatively unfavorable conditions of those areas.

On the other hand, the dominance of corn and soybeans in, say, Iowa does not mean that other crops cannot be grown there. Wheat, potatoes, sugar beets and several other species could be substituted for corn and soybeans, but under present conditions they would be less successful economically. The current need for those commodities is met by production in other areas, even though the yields are sometimes lower than they would be in Iowa.

The assessment of risk and return thus has a great deal to do with the behavior of agricultural systems. The problems are simplified when the farmer centers his operation around a proved low-risk system. Frequently the task requires minimizing diversity. With only a few crops the farmer can acquire through experience and education a great deal of competence for dealing with the or-

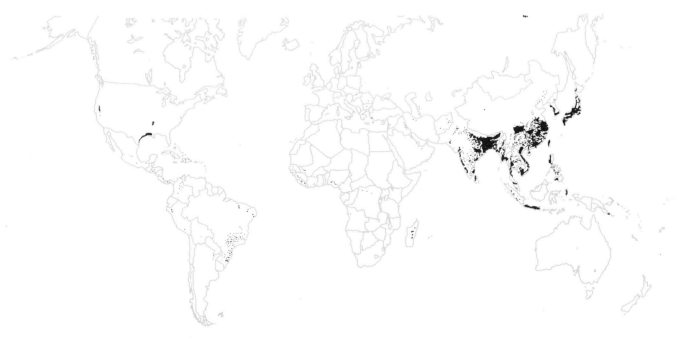

PRODUCTION OF RICE is centered mainly in Asia, but the crop is also grown in a number of other areas that are warm and have good supplies of moisture. Each dot represents 45,000 metric tons; the world total is 300 million metric tons (660 billion pounds) per year.

72   ROBERT S. LOOMIS

dinary adversities of the weather, pests and the market. A farmer who attempts to average his risks from weather over a large number of crops invariably encounters only bad weather; some part of the system is now vulnerable no matter what the sequence of weather is, and the farmer's ability to deal with even ordinary adversities is reduced.

Simplified farms, however, are possible only with machines or where labor is cheap. The labor-intensive farms of India and other developing countries are likely to be quite diversified. The need for labor is thereby distributed more evenly, reducing the peak requirements. Moreover, a greater diversity of food is desirable in subsistence farming. On the other hand, the risk from weather and other problems is high even though it is averaged over several crops. In general, spatial diversification (raising the same crop in different regions) as practiced by industrial farms in the U.S. and Australia is a safer strategy than enterprise diversification (raising many crops in the same environment).

Risk factors can be significantly modified through technology. A basic approach has been to improve the level of environmental tolerance (as by increasing the resistance of a species to pests) through plant breeding. Irrigation systems, tractors, artificial dryers and pest-control agents can have similar effects.

At the same time technologies that can reduce risk may also be employed to enhance income in other ways while leaving the risk at the same level as before. For example, an oversize tractor provides insurance against a wet spring by shortening the time it takes to prepare land for planting, but it can also be used to farm more land with the same amount of labor. Similarly, a grain dryer installed to meet the occasional hazard of cold, wet conditions at the time when standard varieties of grain mature can be applied every year to longer-season varieties that have a higher yield.

The factors that determine agricultural yield are complex. Contrary to a widely held opinion, however, the photosynthetic ability of the plants is seldom a factor, since nutrients, moisture and temperature usually limit the growth of plants to only a fraction of their photosynthetic potential. Plant nutrition in particular presents serious questions for the future of agriculture—probably more serious in the long run than climatic change and other events that might affect agriculture on a large scale. Over a period of time the production rate of stable, well-established agricultural systems will come to equilibrium with the rate of supply of nutrients.

The supply of inorganic nutrients has several sources. Nutrients from the oceans, where salt spray mixes with the atmosphere, are recycled to the land in rainwater. Nutrients are also redistributed on land by transfers of atmospheric dust, by irrigation and by floodwaters. Rice grown in the paddies of Asia, for example, depends significantly on the nutrients leached naturally from upland soils and transported by streams.

The major source of nutrients, however, is the mineral supply of the soil. The supply varies with the type of soil, which is the basic reason for the large differences in fertility between temperate and tropical soils. The differences are related to the conditions of temperature and moisture under which parent materials are weathered and secondary minerals are formed. In addition the young soils of glacial origin in temperate regions have a larger supply of nutrients than the highly leached, senile soils of the Tropics. The most fertile soils in the Tropics are relatively young ones derived from alluvial deposits or volcanic ash. For the world as a whole the area of young and highly fertile soil is quite small.

At present the chief limiting nutrient in agriculture is nitrogen. Given their high capacity for photosynthesis, crop plants in many situations could utilize far more nitrogen than they are likely to receive from natural sources. For example, corn and sugar beets grown in good environments will assimilate more than 500 kilograms of nitrogen per hectare into biomass. The record for annual production of biomass by any plant (a tropical grass that yielded more than 80 tons of dry matter per hectare) involved the assimilation of more than 1,600 kilograms of nitrogen. If a crop is to achieve maximum production, amounts of nitrogen on this order must become available during a single growing season.

Usually the only way to supply nitrogen in such amounts is with fertilizer. An older method, which is less satisfactory from the viewpoint of supplying nitrogen, is to plant legumes, which can fix nitrogen and not only will supply their own needs but also will leave a surplus for subsequent crops. Legumes, however, are rather low-yielding as crops, and the amount of nitrogen they leave in the soil is usually small. Moreover, the fixation of nitrogen by a legume system is

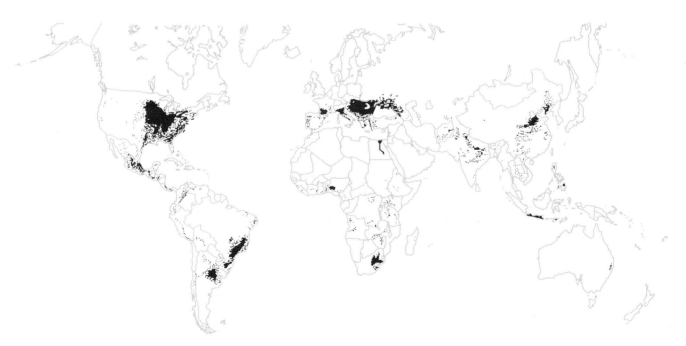

OUTPUT OF CORN is predominantly in the U.S., which accounts for nearly half of the world's production, but the crop also flourishes in many other areas with ample water and a 120-day warm season. Each dot represents 25,000 metric tons; annual total is 300 million.

repressed in the high-nitrogen environments needed for maximum yields of efficient crops such as corn. Under these conditions legumes become net consumers of nitrogen. With the advent in the 1950's of ammonia fertilizers derived from petroleum sources the reliance on legumes as rotation crops has declined.

Agriculture around the world is currently in a state of uncertainty regarding its dependence on legume rotation in the future. As long as new supplies of oil and gas can be found the main reliance is likely to be on fertilizer, even in the poorer countries. The danger with putting additional land into food crops and of emphasizing higher yields is that human populations might expand beyond the level that could be sustained on natural sources of nitrogen alone.

A view of rice production in Indonesia as a system will help to put this problem in focus. In 1972 two crops of rice per year from 10 million hectares of paddy supplied 21 million metric tons of grain, or about 160 kilograms per capita. The harvest represented about 70 percent of the energy and 100 percent of the protein required by the population of 130 million.

The yield, however, was only slightly more than 1,000 kilograms per hectare for each crop of rice, or only 10 percent of the maximum yields of rice established in similar environments and 20 percent of the average yield for Japan and California. The discrepancy is due not so much to a deficiency of human effort (since the standards maintained in Indonesia in such matters as the control of water and weeds are high) as to differences in plant nutrition.

Assuming that the system is in a steady state, a simple nitrogen budget indicates that about 40 kilograms of nitrogen per hectare is removed from the land each year in grain and straw. Even if all the chemical nitrogen consumed in Indonesia were applied to rice land, it would account for only 11 kilograms per hectare of the supply. Legume rotation is not practiced much in Indonesia and rainfall contributes only about 10 kilograms of nitrogen per hectare per year, so that about 19 kilograms must have been supplied through irrigation, manure and fixation by free-living microorganisms. Since it was also necessary to compensate for losses through leaching and denitrification, the amount of nitrogen actually obtained from those sources must have been greater than 19 kilograms and thus close to the maximum amount thought to be available from them.

The point of this exercise is twofold: it reveals the vulnerability of the system to a deficiency in the supply of nitrogen as the level fluctuates from year to year and it shows the enormous potential for

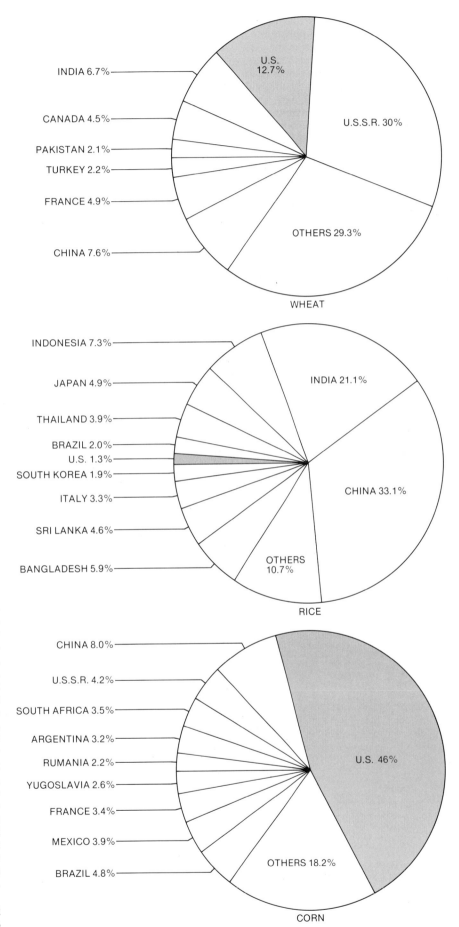

SHARE OF PRODUCTION of wheat, rice and corn by the nations principally involved in growing those crops is charted. The figures represent each major producer's contribution to the annual harvest of the crop. Data were assembled by the U.S. Department of Agriculture.

increases in production. With more nitrogen and an additional supply of other nutrients a fivefold increase in the yield of agricultural crops appears feasible.

The comparison of rice yields in Japan and Indonesia illustrates the wide range in the productivity of agriculture in different regions and different years. There are basically two sources of this variation. One involves differences in climate and other natural factors; the other relates to differences in farm management and the intensity of production.

The effects of natural factors can be strongly modified by the type of technology employed in farm management. If lack of moisture is a problem, for example, marked increases in yield per planted hectare can be obtained by leaving a field fallow every other year. Irrigation provides even greater increases.

The type and amount of technology employed are a function of current markets and the social system. Different resources are optimized in different systems. Indonesia is clearly tending to optimize a scarce resource associated with

land: the natural supply of nutrients. Japan optimizes the amount of sunlight by supplying nutrients to achieve a high yield per unit of area. Similar strategies are employed in Israel and the Netherlands. Such land-poor countries provide a practical definition of intensive agriculture, namely how close the level of production is brought to the potential offered by biology and climate.

The agriculture of the U.S. is of intermediate intensity. One might suppose the extensive reliance on machinery in the U.S. indicates highly intensive farming, but machinery by itself is not an indicator of intensity. Although some intensification is achieved with mechanization (for example, through a better seedbed and a more timely harvest), yields can also be lowered when wide spacing of rows is required to accommodate machines and when the operation of machines compacts the soil. What the machine-oriented agriculture of the U.S. reflects is the optimization of labor in a social environment where land, energy and capital are relatively cheap.

The lower end of the scale of intensifi-

cation is characterized by the agriculture of much of Asia and Africa. There the yield of grain is typically in the range from 700 to 1,400 kilograms per hectare. Many of these farming systems are very old, and some of them are rather finely tuned. External inputs such as fertilizer and machinery are low. The systems represent a type of ecological steady state that might be sustained indefinitely. Provided that the level of human population is held within the capability of the system, these systems are probably as safe as any that could be devised. The intensive systems are also relatively safe, provided that they receive maintenance, research and high priorities for land and energy. Their stability is thus determined to a large extent by factors outside the farming system.

All these systems are highly responsive to market conditions. Production that cannot be channeled to markets directly or through livestock has little value to society. One result is that production is strongly constrained to match demand. Management decisions on the quality and amount of land given to each crop, on the varieties of crop, on the uses made of the crop and on the level of farming effort make it possible for the level of effective output to be varied over a considerable range.

In many cases the disincentives to increased production are greatest in societies that appear to have the greatest need for it. To satisfy urban needs many developing nations have found it necessary to maintain policies favoring a low cost for food and thus a low return to farmers. It has been possible to take this course because the food markets of the world have been depressed for 100 years by the abundant production of American agriculture.

One result of the effects of social factors is that little can be deduced about the potential behavior of a farming system by examining its present performance, unless the inquiry is focused on matters of biology, soil and climate. Considering only such natural factors, one can say that with the present base of arable land, with a largely vegetarian diet based on yields that could be achieved with present knowledge and with a substantial amount of energy and human effort the world could support a human population of 50 billion or more. The food system would be heavily dependent, however, on the smooth functioning of the larger society. The Irish famine of the 1840's, for example, was more a failure of human institutions than of biology. Biology and climate will vary, and adjustments take time. Even a moderately intensive farming system such as the one in the U.S. requires constant attention to genetic resources and the supply of energy. The benign neglect of agriculture as one of the lesser pursuits of man is no longer possible.

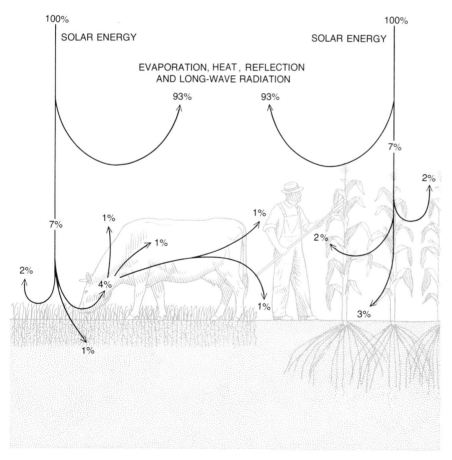

PARTITIONING OF ENERGY involved in producing such crops as corn and grass is depicted. Of the solar energy that reaches the earth at a rate of 500 calories per square centimeter per day about 93 percent returns to the atmosphere. With nutrients and water abundant and with a full cover of leaves about 7 percent of solar energy can be converted in photosynthesis; 2 percent goes into respiration, which is required for the growth and maintenance of the crop, and 5 percent goes into the dry matter of the crop. In corn 3 percent goes into roots, stems and leaves, which constitute a crop residue that is recycled to the soil or fed to animals, and 2 percent emerges as grain directly edible by man. For grass as much as 4 percent may be consumed by the cow. The energy represented by the food consumed by human beings and animals is further broken down for both the cow and the corn crop in the manner indicated by the diagram.

7

The Agriculture of the U.S.

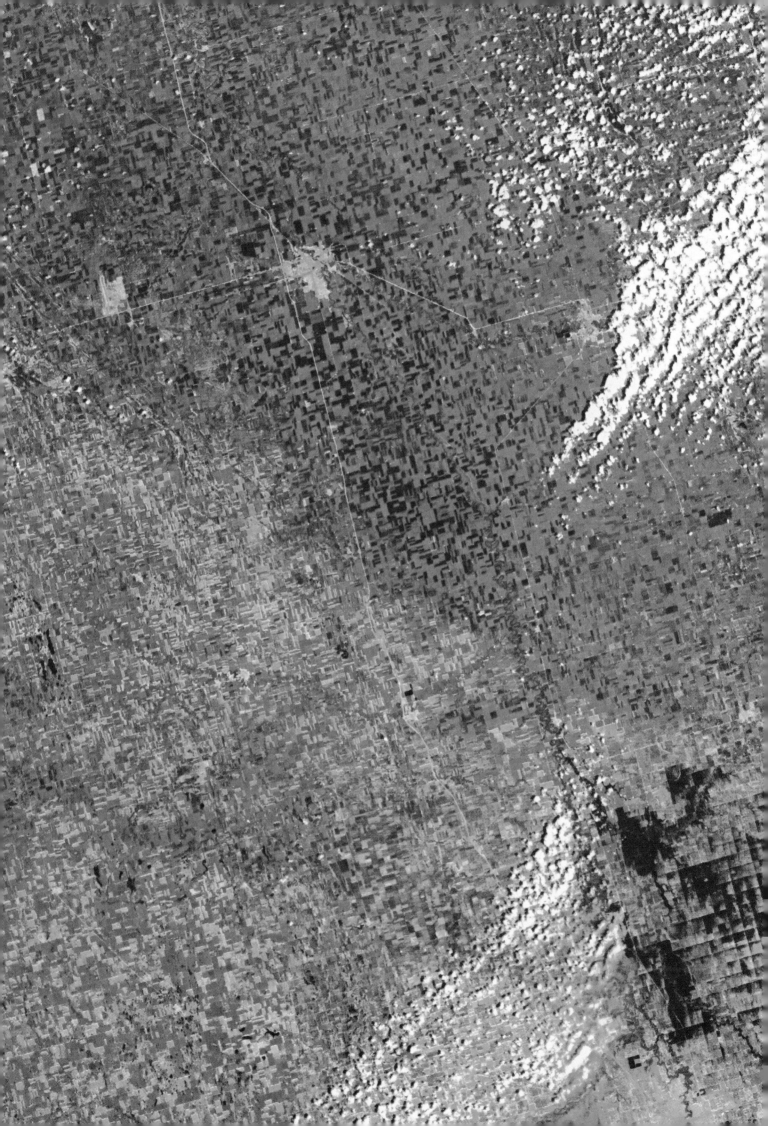

The Agriculture of the U. S.

EARL O. HEADY

Its high productivity is a result of two centuries of development policy: low prices for land and other things needed for farming, stable prices for farm products and the promotion of innovation.

The agriculture of the U.S. currently plays a vital and unique role in the economy of both the nation and the world. In the nation the agricultural sector has enjoyed high profits during the past three years when most other sectors of the economy were experiencing a recession and a decline in income. Employment in agriculture remained quite stable, even though elsewhere in the economy the rate of unemployment greatly increased. Moreover, the secular trend of workers migrating out of agricultural jobs as a result of technological change in agriculture has recently slackened. Over the past several years capital assets, particularly land, have sharply increased in value to record levels. In contrast, the value of corporate bonds and common stocks were strongly depressed during much of the same period. Even during the worldwide recession from 1973 through 1975 the dollar value of farm exports rose to an annual average level of $18.5 billion, an annual increase of 167 percent over the period between 1968 and 1972. Agricultural exports have accounted for a growing portion of the nation's foreign exchange and have played an important role in creating for the U.S. a positive balance of trade.

In the economy of the world American agriculture dominated food exports. Between 1973 and 1975 grain exports from the U.S. accounted for 65 percent of the world's total grain exports. The importance of American agriculture in solving world food problems is obvious. Currently the product of nearly one in every five crop acres in the U.S. is ex-

ported, and the output of a full 14 percent of our farm work force moves into world markets. Yet agriculture employs only 5 percent of the labor force in the U.S., and only 4.4 percent of the nation's population. No other important food-producing country of large population approaches the U.S. in the degree to which it has reduced its farm labor force. It is the great productivity of American agriculture that enables the nation to acquire its food with minimal labor.

How did American agriculture attain such world supremacy in productivity? Has the agricultural sector in the U.S. reached the limits of its productive capacity, or can that capacity be further increased? Can the keys to such productivity be transported to other countries? What future economic and social problems, if any, are in store for the agricultural sector in the U.S.? How would such problems affect rural communities and other segments of the society?

Agricultural economists and other agricultural specialists in the U.S. have been probing the world of the developing countries over the past two decades to find the key to successful agricultural development. They need not have traveled so far; the secrets of successful agricultural development are best found in the past history of the U.S.

Over the past 200 years the U.S. has had the best, the most logical and the most successful program of agricultural development anywhere in the world. Other countries would do well to copy it. Although the program was put to-

gether piecemeal over many decades, by and large instruments of policy were consciously devised to encourage the agricultural sector to expand its resources and increase its output. As a result of such conscious policy the consumer in the U.S., and to a lesser extent in the rest of the world, has realized a favorable price for food. By 1971 only 15.7 percent of the disposable income of the average American consumer was spent for food. (In 1975 that figure rose to 16.8 percent because of inflation.) By way of comparison, in developing countries in 1971 the average consumer spent 65 percent of his disposable income for food, in the U.S.S.R. he spent 30 percent and in the countries of the European Economic Community he spent 26 percent.

What are the specific elements of a successful and conscious agricultural development policy? First, the policy must enlarge the farmer's supply of major resources and keep their prices low. Second, it must keep the prices of the commodities produced on the farm relatively high and stable. Third, it must create a tenure system that structures the operating costs of the farms in a way that is favorable to innovation. Fourth, it must encourage research and technology, and it must maintain an adequate and continuous flow of information to the farmer on the availability of new techniques and technology. The U.S. has implemented all these elements in its agricultural development policy, sometimes separately, usually in combination with one another. Over the decades the specific methods by which the Government has implemented its agricultural policy have changed, but the general principle of encouraging agricultural development has remained the same.

At the beginning of the nation's agricultural development land was abundant and labor was cheap. Capital inputs such as farm machinery, fertilizer and food for the farmer's family were relatively modest, and most of them were produced on the farm. Farmers created their own power in the form of the physical work of family members

LARGE RECTANGULAR FIELDS, aligned predominantly along north-south east-west axes, make up the characteristic pattern of agriculture in the Great Plains region of the U.S., represented on the opposite page by a digitally processed LANDSAT 2 image recorded on July 5, 1975. The scene encompasses a portion of the Red River Valley near the border between North Dakota and Minnesota. The large blue area at upper left near intersection of two major highways is the town of Grand Forks, N.D. In the false-color scheme used to make this picture the red areas are crops under cultivation, the blue areas are land lying fallow, the black areas are water remaining after a recent flood and the irregular white patches are clouds. Heavily flooded area at lower right is crisscrossed by roads delineating section lines. Principal crops under cultivation when the picture was made were wheat, potatoes and sugar beets.

and of animals raised on the farm. They also harnessed energy from the sun for that work in the form of crops grown on the farm and eaten by the people or the animals. The farmers generated their own fertilizer by rotating crops and by utilizing the wastes from the animals. The rotation of crops also controlled insects to some extent.

Because of the availability of land farms expanded rapidly across the nation. The growth in their output could be readily absorbed by the market. The demand for food was quite elastic because of the steady increase in population, in per capita income and in food exports. Food-marketing facilities also expanded through public policies that provided land grants to railroad builders. With the markets growing and the demand for food increasing, the agricultural policy was predominantly a developmental one emphasizing large supplies of major farm resources and low prices for them. In general, the nation's development policy for agriculture benefited farmers through low property values (and therefore low land costs) and high income, and it simultaneously benefited consumers with favorable real prices for food.

American agricultural policy in the 19th century was certainly the most successful policy for development the world had yet seen. After the U.S. had expanded to the Pacific and the public domain for land grants was exhausted, the Government did not terminate the agricultural development policy. It simply shifted its emphasis. Instead of concentrating on expansion it began to emphasize productivity. It turned to scientific knowledge and new technology as capital resources to be supplied either at low cost or free. The Morrill Act of 1862 created the land-grant college system to encourage research and to extend new technical knowledge to farmers. The new resources were an effective substitute for land: between 1910 and 1970 the output of American agriculture approximately doubled; furthermore, by 1970 the nation was producing its food on considerably fewer acres than it had been in 1910, and production-control programs were in effect. The results of public investment in technical improvement in agriculture were particularly apparent after 1940 as research became more refined and systematic. Moreover, the technologies incorporated into the new farming practices were low in cost compared with the quantity of agricultural products to which they gave rise. Hence the new capital technologies were adopted rapidly, and by the 1950's they became an effective substitute not only for land but also for labor. The result was that between 1950 and 1955 more than a million workers migrated out of the agricultural sector into other sectors of the economy.

Other Government development policies also helped to increase the supply of resources for agriculture and thereby reduce their cost. The Federal Farm Loan Act of 1916 and subsequent legislation provided publicly supported means whereby farmers could obtain capital assets such as farm machinery at lower interest rates than those prevailing in the open market. Similarly, the National Reclamation Act of 1902 provided means by which semiarid land in the West was supplied to farmers at subsidized prices to encourage them to develop it through irrigation.

The nation's development policy for agriculture has been implemented vigorously over most of the past 200 years. It is still in force. It is reflected in publicly supported research, education, farm credits and other programs that develop new capital technologies and encourage their exploitation by farmers. The development policy for agriculture in the U.S. is a landmark example to which the governments of developing nations might pay heed as they struggle to raise their food production above the level of subsistence.

A nation can rely on a development

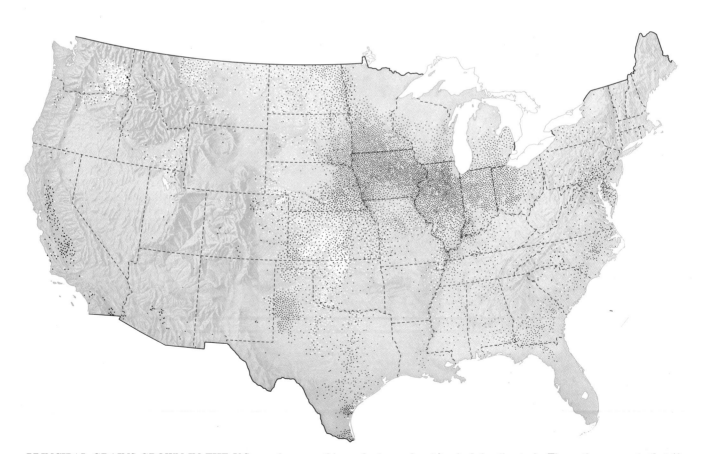

PRINCIPAL GRAINS GROWN IN THE U.S. are shown on this outline map of the nation. The dots in white represent acreage devoted to wheat raised for human consumption. The dots in black represent acreage devoted to the major feed grains (corn, grain sorghum, barley and oats) raised for livestock. The author suggests that if American consumers reduced their meat intake by 25 percent, and if silage were substituted for 25 percent of the grain fed to livestock, American grain exports to poor countries could more than double.

policy to simultaneously benefit farmers and consumers only when the demand for food is both elastic and growing. Although that was the case in the U.S. until early in the 20th century, by the 1920's the per capita income had risen high enough for the domestic demand for food to have become highly inelastic. That is, incomes had risen to the level where consumers were able to buy all the food they needed and further increases in income could have little effect on food consumption. The result of such inelasticity is that an increase in food output of 1 percent leads to a decrease in food prices of more than 1 percent. If other factors, such as exports, remain at constant levels, an increase in farm production greater than the rate of population growth causes the market price of food to decline at a rate greater than the growth of demand. The total real market revenue from agricultural products thus declines.

Such a decline began in the 1920's and was intensified by the Great Depression of the 1930's. It was relieved during World War II and the period of postwar reconstruction, when the U.S. exported food to countries whose agricultural production had been disrupted by the war. By 1950, however, world agricultural production had recovered. Again the market situation for U.S. farm commodities was one of highly inelastic demand both at home and abroad. The conditions of the 1920's had returned. Agricultural development and greater farm output alone could no longer guarantee gains simultaneously to both farmers and consumers because the benefits and the costs of continued development were inequitably distributed. As farm output continued to grow, the consumers were benefited by lower real prices for food but the farmers suffered from a decline in income.

To counteract the effects of inelastic demand agricultural policy in the U.S. took yet another course. It began providing a series of compensatory programs to maintain farm income at acceptable levels. Farmers were paid to reduce their planted acreage and output. Their reduced output supported higher prices of food on the market. Farmers were also lent money and storage facilities in ways such that the rate at which their products were put on the market was controlled. Furthermore, international food-aid programs were devised to subsidize exports—sometimes in effect giving produce away—both to help increase the demand for food and to encourage developing countries to accept it. Such programs, financed by the public through taxes during the 1930's and again from the 1950's through 1972, were compensatory in two senses. First, the programs directly paid farmers to compensate them for reductions in their income from the market as the supply of food increased more rapidly than the demand. Second, by controlling farm production the programs offset or compensated for the greater productivity of farms that had been promoted through agricultural research, soil conservation, irrigation and other development efforts.

After the 1930's, then, the U.S. had in operation both development programs and compensatory programs. The compensatory programs did not totally offset or eliminate the effects of the development programs. As agriculture continued to improve its technology the programs controlling the supply of food to the market served only to slow the growth of farm output, not to stop it. Between 1950 and 1972 the price of new capital technologies remained favorable with respect to the moderate market prices of produce, and agricultural productivity continued to advance. Farms

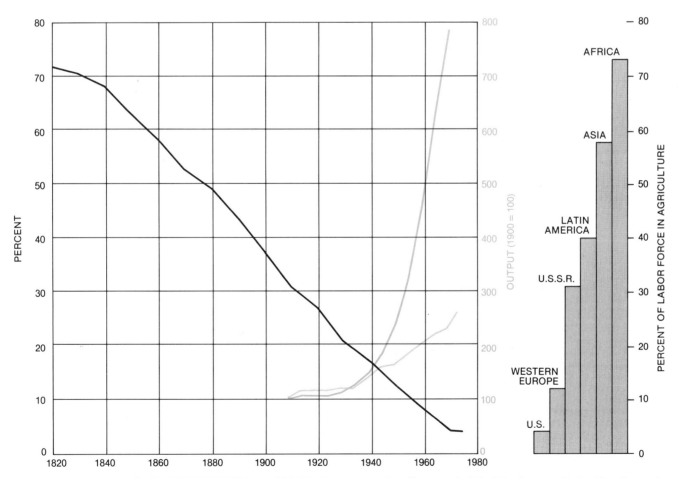

PERCENT OF LABOR FORCE ON THE LAND in the U.S. (*black*) has declined steadily over the past 150 years (*left*). Yet between 1910 and 1970 the absolute output of farms has approximately doubled (*light color*). Moreover, the productivity of American farms per farm worker has increased enormously (*dark color*). For the purposes of comparison the percent of the labor force on the land in other parts of the world is shown by the bar graph at the right. The percentages are averages for very large areas and conceal such information as the fact that 7 percent of the labor force of Israel is engaged in agriculture, whereas 91 percent of the labor force of Chad is so engaged.

became larger and more specialized, handling either crops or livestock instead of both. Farms growing crops greatly increased their utilization of fertilizers, pesticides, farm machinery and other capital items. For example, the use of fertilizer increased by 276 percent between 1950 and 1972. The use of powered machines increased by only 30 percent, but in 1972 there were substantially fewer farms than there were in 1950, and the average farm was more highly mechanized than its counterpart in 1950. The result was that farm labor declined by 54 percent over that period as labor productivity quadrupled and total farm output increased by 55 percent.

The compensatory programs called for large outlays of funds, and by the 1960's the public was spending heavily. By 1968 the total cost of the programs was $5.7 billion per year, and by 1972 it had reached $7 billion. More than a third of all the wheat grown in the U.S. was exported in 1965, and more than a fourth of it was exported in 1970. Other exports subsidized under foreign food-aid programs were feed grains, rice, tobacco and milk. The decade beginning with 1970 hence appeared at the outset to be a continuation of the 1950's and 1960's.

No one, however, could have fore-seen the failure of the Russian wheat crop in 1972. As a result between 1971 and 1972 American wheat exports almost doubled. Feed-grain exports also grew. With the failure of the Peruvian anchovy catch in 1973 and 1974, and the consequent protein shortage in areas that relied on the anchovies as a feed supplement, in 1973 American exports of protein-rich soybeans more than doubled over those in 1971.

With such high export levels the prices of farm commodities rose sharply. Furthermore, American crops showed record yields in both 1974 and 1975. Thus farm income also attained record levels. The rapid upward movement in income has put farmers in a highly favorable position with regard to capital assets. Although some farmers took advantage of the opportunity to repay their mortgage before it came due, the majority put their higher earnings into acquiring new farm equipment, upgrading their living facilities and enlarging their farms by buying more land. As a result farm real estate values more than doubled between 1970 and 1975.

The supply-control programs were eliminated early in 1974. Hence for the past three years U.S. agriculture has been operating in a free market.

Although the compensatory pro-grams have held farm incomes at acceptable levels, they have had an adverse effect on some groups and conditions off the farm, an effect that has not been lessened even though the programs have been discontinued. The change in the very nature of farming, with its higher productivity and greater degree of mechanization, has severely affected rural communities in agricultural areas. With the decline in the farm population the demand for the goods and services of businesses in country towns has been eroded. Employment and income opportunities in typical rural communities have therefore declined markedly. As people migrated out of the rural communities, there were fewer people left to participate in the services of schools, medical facilities and other institutions. With the lessened demand such services retreated in quantity and quality and advanced in cost.

Nonfarm groups in the rural communities took large capital losses as country businesses closed down and their operators moved elsewhere, in many cases leaving their dwellings to decay. Although the compensatory programs helped to prevent farms from losing their income, there were no similar programs for other enterprises in rural areas.

Rapid agricultural development in

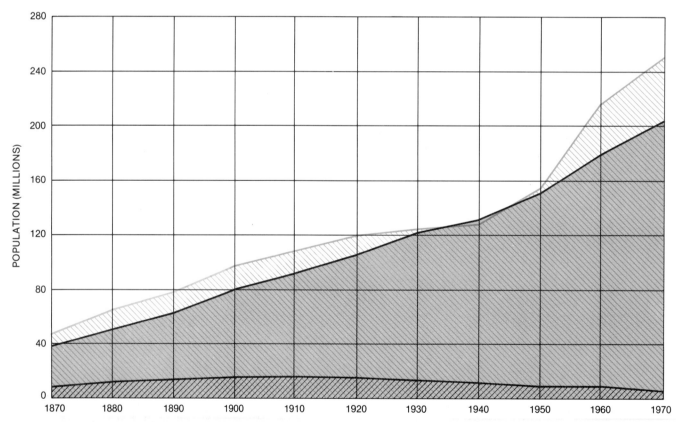

PRODUCTIVITY OF AMERICAN AGRICULTURE has been high for most of the past 100 years as a result of the agricultural policy in the U.S. The gray area represents the total population of the U.S. at 10-year intervals from 1870 through 1970. The black hatched area shows the number of workers in agriculture for the same period. The colored hatched area shows the number of people those American **farm workers could feed. Although the absolute number of people on the land in 1970 was approximately half the number of people on the land in 1870, the productivity per worker was 10 times greater in 1970. Currently American agriculture can feed about 50 million more people than live in the country, and some 20 percent of all farm produce is exported. The limits of productivity have not been reached.**

the U.S. in recent decades has also had a heavy impact on the environment. Farms have become larger and more specialized in crops such as wheat, corn and soybeans, depleting the soil of certain specific nutrients and thus requiring larger amounts of fertilizer. As Government supply-control programs curtailed the areas planted to crops in the 1950's and 1960's, farmers cultivated their remaining land more intensively and applied even larger quantities of fertilizers and pesticides. The burden placed on streams and lakes by the runoff of silt and farm chemicals therefore increased.

On the other hand, the development of American agriculture has fostered the growth of an entire agricultural industry—"agribusiness"—of which farming is only a small part. The modern agricultural industry has three ma-

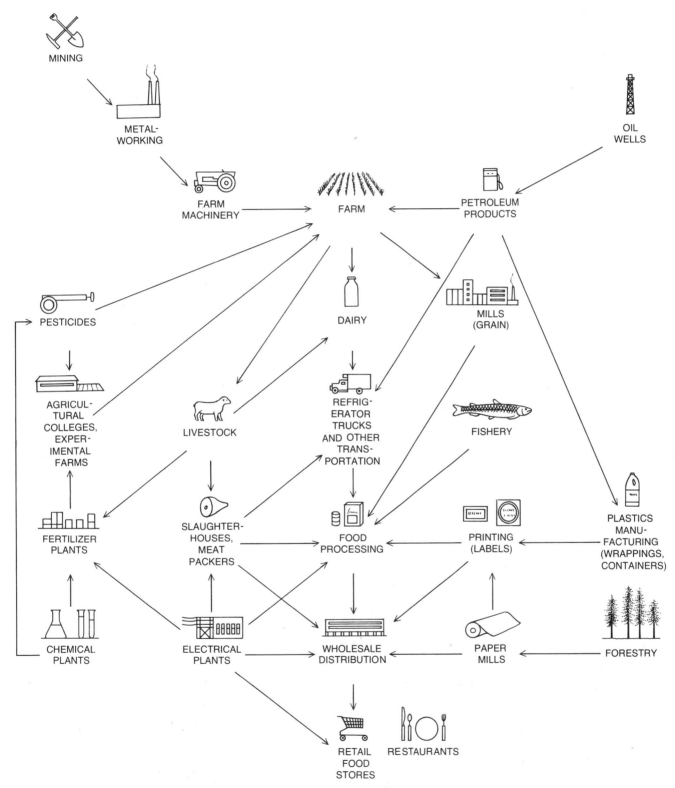

THE "AGRIBUSINESS," or entire food industry of the U.S., is intricately interwoven with many sectors of the economy and encompasses far more than farming. The flow chart gives a visual impression of the interaction of farming and other activities. On the input side of the farm are industries that supply such items as farm machinery and fertilizer; on the output side of the farm is the food-processing industry. Input-output chart on page 82 shows the interaction of farming and industry in greater detail in terms of sums of money.

	FOOD AND KINDRED PRODUCTS	LIVESTOCK AND LIVESTOCK PRODUCTS	OTHER AGRICULTURAL PRODUCTS	AGRICULTURAL, FORESTRY AND FISHERY SERVICES	PERSONAL CONSUMPTION EXPENDITURES	NET INVENTORY CHANGE	NET EXPORTS	FEDERAL GOVERNMENT PURCHASES	STATE AND LOCAL GOVERNMENT PURCHASES	TOTAL GROSS PRIVATE FIXED CAPITAL FORMATION	TOTAL FINAL DEMAND	TOTAL OUTPUT
AGRICULTURAL PRODUCTS												
FOOD AND KINDRED PRODUCTS	17,212	4,053	—	39	71,970	732	2,423	467	734	—	76,325	105,045
LIVESTOCK AND LIVESTOCK PRODUCTS	23,466	7,390	1,581	185	2,321	698	68	6	23	—	3,116	37,504
OTHER AGRICULTURAL PRODUCTS	7,564	9,468	935	559	4,161	118	3,562	-1,106	129	—	6,864	30,195
AGRICULTURAL, FORESTRY AND FISHERY SERVICES	—	610	1,341	—	240	—	19	10	45	—	314	2,899
BUILDING AND MAINTENANCE												
NEW CONSTRUCTION	535	514	809	33	—	—	22	3,290	24,806	68,601	96,719	96,719
MAINTENANCE AND REPAIR CONSTRUCTION	352	233	358	—	—	—	—	1,499	5,280	—	6,780	30,999
MACHINERY												
FARM MACHINERY	1	70	2,685	102	43	221	393	26	44	2,928	3,656	4,756
MATERIALS-HANDLING MACHINERY AND EQUIPMENT	144	—	—	—	—	28	204	78	1	1,440	1,751	3,073
SPECIAL-INDUSTRY MACHINERY AND EQUIPMENT	560	—	—	13	32	60	1,124	44	16	3,538	4,813	6,353
MOTOR VEHICLES AND OTHER TRANSPORTATION EQUIPMENT	199	416	515	10	17,621	-304	3,068	2,451	1,252	15,558	39,644	57,799
OFFICE, COMPUTING AND ACCOUNTING MACHINES	92	2	1	3	111	152	1,578	648	219	4,195	6,902	9,297
SERVICE-INDUSTRY MACHINES	93	18	2	2	548	176	512	92	170	2,087	3,585	6,895
MISCELLANEOUS ELECTRICAL MACHINES, EQUIPMENT AND SUPPLIES	7	15	45	—	791	87	228	128	43	268	1,544	3,945
PROFESSIONAL, SCIENTIFIC, CONTROL, OPTICAL, PHOTOGRAPHIC INSTRUMENTS, EQUIPMENT SUPPLIES	89	—	3	6	1,845	194	1,180	1,207	481	2,530	7,437	12,993
FERTILIZERS AND CHEMICALS												
CHEMICAL AND FERTILIZER MINERAL MINING	4	—	10	—	3	10	114	—	88	—	213	924
CHEMICALS AND SELECTED CHEMICAL PRODUCTS	458	92	2,274	17	601	282	2,294	1,606	234	—	5,017	26,245
ENERGY												
PETROLEUM REFINING AND RELATED INDUSTRIES	250	192	942	5	12,271	353	950	963	463	—	15,000	31,765
ELECTRIC, GAS, WATER AND SANITARY SERVICES	740	113	247	2	17,676	—	84	449	2,571	—	20,781	47,871
CONTAINERS												
MISCELLANEOUS TEXTILE GOODS AND FLOOR COVERINGS	20	11	29	45	1,814	11	98	19	1	123	2,066	5,573
MISCELLANEOUS FABRICATED TEXTILE PRODUCTS	90	*	45	4	2,497	117	72	299	32	—	3,017	5,034
PLASTICS AND SYNTHETIC MATERIALS	90	—	—	—	21	84	834	58	1	—	998	10,158
RUBBER AND MISCELLANEOUS PLASTICS PRODUCTS	793	45	188	*	3,172	329	416	303	275	29	4,523	17,213
GLASS AND GLASS PRODUCTS	1,329	6	—	—	443	100	189	18	82	—	832	4,768
METAL CONTAINERS	2,645	19	12	—	—	124	15	11	—	11	161	4,490
LUMBER AND WOOD PRODUCTS (EXCEPT CONTAINERS)	12	4	4	—	401	163	612	29	5	8	1,217	15,330
WOODEN CONTAINERS	96	—	80	8	—	2	3	22	—	—	26	456
PAPER AND ALLIED PRODUCTS (EXCEPT CONTAINERS AND BOXES)	950	17	1	*	1,907	179	1,013	115	283	—	3,498	19,769
PAPERBOARD CONTAINERS AND BOXES	1,916	2	3	117	87	40	27	32	29	—	215	7,051
SERVICES												
OFFICE SUPPLIES	72	1	1	*	—	—	—	174	442	—	616	3,266
PRINTING AND PUBLISHING	579	9	14	*	5,113	113	289	213	1,134	—	6,862	26,002
TRANSPORTATION AND WAREHOUSING	3,243	874	597	31	14,015	289	4,987	2,960	1,419	967	24,636	65,679
COMMUNICATIONS, EXCEPT BROADCASTING	374	96	85	—	10,400	—	320	665	752	1,655	13,791	25,645
WHOLESALE AND RETAIL TRADE	4,347	1,731	2,666	76	140,630	516	2,984	1,108	727	7,808	153,773	207,109
FINANCE AND INSURANCE	494	379	432	3	31,359	—	169	57	621	16	32,221	65,495
REAL ESTATE AND RENTAL	908	581	2,402	80	89,935	—	811	337	1,052	2,567	94,701	143,163
HOTELS AND LODGING PLACES, PERSONAL AND REPAIR SERVICES (EXCEPT AUTOMOBILE REPAIRS)	164	6	—	—	17,741	—	8	568	185	—	18,501	23,636
BUSINESS SERVICES	3,752	95	1,385	*	6,291	—	485	2,491	2,391	—	11,658	68,991
AUTOMOBILE REPAIR AND SERVICES	227	155	159	1	10,248	—	—	49	240	—	10,536	18,443
BUSINESS TRAVEL, ENTERTAINMENT AND GIFTS	414	32	44	13	—	—	—	—	—	—	—	13,324
VALUE ADDED	27,650	10,772	14,311	1,700	—	—	—	—	—	—	—	973,114

jor components. The first is the input-processing industry that produces the seed, machines, fertilizers, pesticides, fuel and other things needed for large-scale farming. The second component is the farm itself, which consumes the inputs in the raising of crops and animals. The third component is the food-processing industry, which takes over the products of farms, transports them to processing centers where they are cooked, canned, frozen, dehydrated, reconstituted, wrapped and labeled, and then distributes them to wholesale and retail outlets.

The input-processing industry now supplies many things that were once produced on the farm. Today tractors substitute for draft animals, fossil fuels for animal feeds, chemical fertilizers for manure and nitrogen-fixing crops. Such developments not only have shifted a greater proportion of the agricultural work force from the farms into the input-processing sector but also have increased the cash cost of farming as a percentage of the total cost. The greater proportion of cash cost has made farm profits much more vulnerable to price fluctuations than they used to be.

The food-processing sector has in recent years come to represent a larger proportion of the total agricultural industry than farming itself. In 1975, 42 cents of each consumer dollar spent for food at retail prices went to the farmer and 58 cents went to the food processors. Even the typical commercial farm family now buys frozen, packaged and ready-to-serve foods from the supermarket rather than consuming products raised and prepared on the farm.

The largest fraction of the cost of processing and handling food between the farm gate and the retail store is for labor, accounting for 51 percent. The remaining 49 percent is divided among the actual processing of the food, materials for packaging the food, transportation, rent, depreciation, promotion, interest, repairs, taxes and other expenses. Those costs will continue to increase as consumers, including farm families, demand an increasing amount of processing and a greater number of services to

go along with their food. The tendency toward higher costs is accelerating as the quick-food industry flourishes and as a greater number of people eat meals away from home.

The change in the nature of agriculture has greatly enhanced the financial position of established farmers with large holdings; for them the period from 1960 through 1975 has been the most profitable period in the history of farming. The situation is not as favorable for farmers who are starting from scratch. Because of inflation in general and the upsurge in land values in particular the amount of capital required to start a new farm is now quite high. Moreover, since established farmers are investing their expanded earnings in increasing their own holdings, beginning farmers or those with only a small amount of capital have difficulty gaining a competitive position. One can therefore expect to see an increasing trend toward more large commercial farms and fewer small ones. In addition a substantial fraction of the older established farmers will soon be retiring and turning their farms over to their children, and this younger generation of established farmers tends to be better educated and to have higher management skills than the older generation.

The large capital assets of the established farms, the increase in their size and the intense competition among them encourages their operators to quickly adopt new and promising technological developments. Hence even with the high cost of energy and chemicals and increasing environmental restraints American agriculture is likely to make a great technological leap forward over the next few years. Such an advance, coupled with the fact that more land is being shifted from pasture and forest to crops, could mean that the productivity of American agriculture will continue to increase in the years ahead.

The future of American agriculture will depend on a number of factors in addition to its productive capacity. The two most important factors will be the extent to which recent international conditions continue to prevail and the presence or absence of Government policies affecting output either through future supply-control programs or environmental limits on fertilizers, pesticides and soil erosion.

It is likely that the rapid rise in the world demand for American grain exports since 1972 has both transitory and permanent elements. The unfavorable weather in the U.S.S.R. and the poor anchovy catch off Peru are transitory elements, intensified by the devaluation of the dollar twice in the early 1970's. The permanent elements are such factors as the continuing upward

trend in world population and per capita income, and the shift toward the consumption of more meat in the developing countries. Such long-term trends are rather smooth; unlike the transitory elements, they are not quantum jumps in the long-term world demand for grain.

There are, of course, many hungry people in the world who would eat more if they had a higher income or were given food on a charitable basis. At the moment, however, there is no prospect that these things will come to pass. Thus the demand for the grain of the U.S. and the other major grain-producing countries will intensify as both the population and the income of the developing countries increase. In some years that gradual upward trend in the world demand for exported grain may be interrupted as crops in other countries do better or worse.

The U.S.S.R. and other countries are concerned to build up grain reserves to protect their consumers from exaggerated swings in food prices. Until effective world grain-reserve facilities are created, however, or unless the U.S. itself reserves great quantities of grains, American agriculture may be affected by whiplash fluctuations in world grain prices, with high and low levels of exports and high and low levels of income. In other words, the prospect for the prices of grain and food is one of great instability.

Such instability is not, however, inevitable. If international organizations or a single world organization could establish institutions that would make added output from American agriculture available to the world's hungry, and if the effort could be made economic for American farmers, the U.S. could increase its agricultural output and exports by a substantial amount over the output and exports of the 1970's. The U.S. has a considerable reserve of land that could be planted to crops if it were profitable to do so. The latest available census data show that in 1969 the nation had 422 million acres of cropland, of which only 333 million acres were devoted to crops; the remainder was given over to pasture or lay fallow. Moreover, the nation has an additional 264 million acres of forest, pasture, rangeland and wetlands, some of which could, if it were essential, be converted to cropland.

If just the unused cropland were now converted to crops, if water were utilized efficiently and if all proved new technologies were adopted, by 1985 the nation could fully meet all domestic demand and still increase its exports of grain by 183 percent over the record average level between 1972 and 1974. Specifically, corn exports could be increased by 228 percent, wheat exports by 57 percent and soybean exports by

INPUT-OUTPUT CHART shows the major sectors of the economy with which American agriculture interacted in 1970. Numbers in boxes are millions of dollars given in terms of the value of the dollar in 1967. Inputs to agriculture are in vertical columns. Output from agriculture to the rest of economy is in horizontal rows. A dash (—) in a box indicates that there was no transaction; an asterisk (*) indicates that transaction was less than $500 thousand. Chart was compiled with help of Anne P. Carter of Brandeis University.

363 percent. Furthermore, if some of the 264 million acres of potential cropland were brought into production, exports by the year 2000 could be even greater.

Grain exports could be increased even without converting any additional land to crops. If American consumers were to substitute soybean protein for only 25 percent of the meat in their diet, less grain would be needed to feed livestock; by 1985 the U.S. could export 80 percent more feed grains, soybeans and wheat than it did between 1971 and 1974. Alternatively, if American consumers reduced their total meat intake by 25 percent, the U.S. could export 103 percent more grain. Or if silage were substituted for 25 percent of the grain that is fed to cattle, American grain exports could be increased by 110 percent. What if all three of those things were done? By 1985 American grain exports could be increased by 135 percent.

To me all of the above suggests that the world's food problems can be brought under control by two main ef-

forts. First, as other authors in this issue of *Scientific American* have emphasized, the governments of the poor countries must actively encourage the development of their own agriculture. Second, since it is unlikely that even with such development all the poor countries will be able to feed themselves for some time to come, world institutions and markets must be created in order to absorb more of the output of the food-exporting countries at prices that are economic for their farmers.

Today the cash cost of farming has risen so high that the break-even prices of farm produce have doubled over what they were in 1970. American farmers are unlikely to risk increasing their output to high levels unless certain base prices are guaranteed. Until such guarantees are adopted, and until worldwide public policies establishing grain reserves against the lean years are in effect, the instability of world grain prices is likely to restrain American farmers from enlarging the amount of land they have under cultivation and increasing their output.

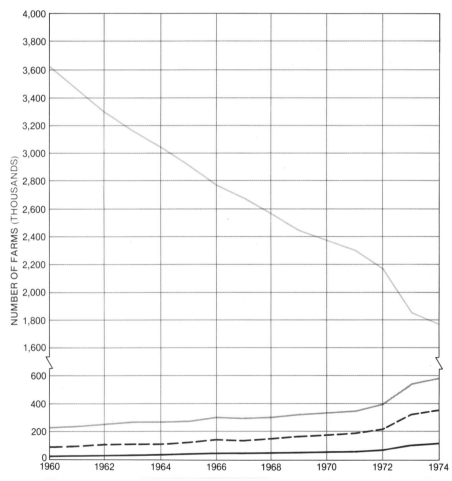

NUMBER OF SMALL FARMS HAS DECREASED between 1960 and 1974 at the same time that the number of large farms has increased. The reason is that cash costs of farming are now so high that farmers without large capital assets are unable to compete with farmers with large holdings. Farms are grouped according to whether they sold more than $100,000 worth of produce per year (*solid black line*), between $40,000 and $99,999 worth (*broken black line*), between $20,000 and $39,999 worth (*gray line*) or less than $20,000 worth (*colored line*).

8

The Agriculture of Mexico

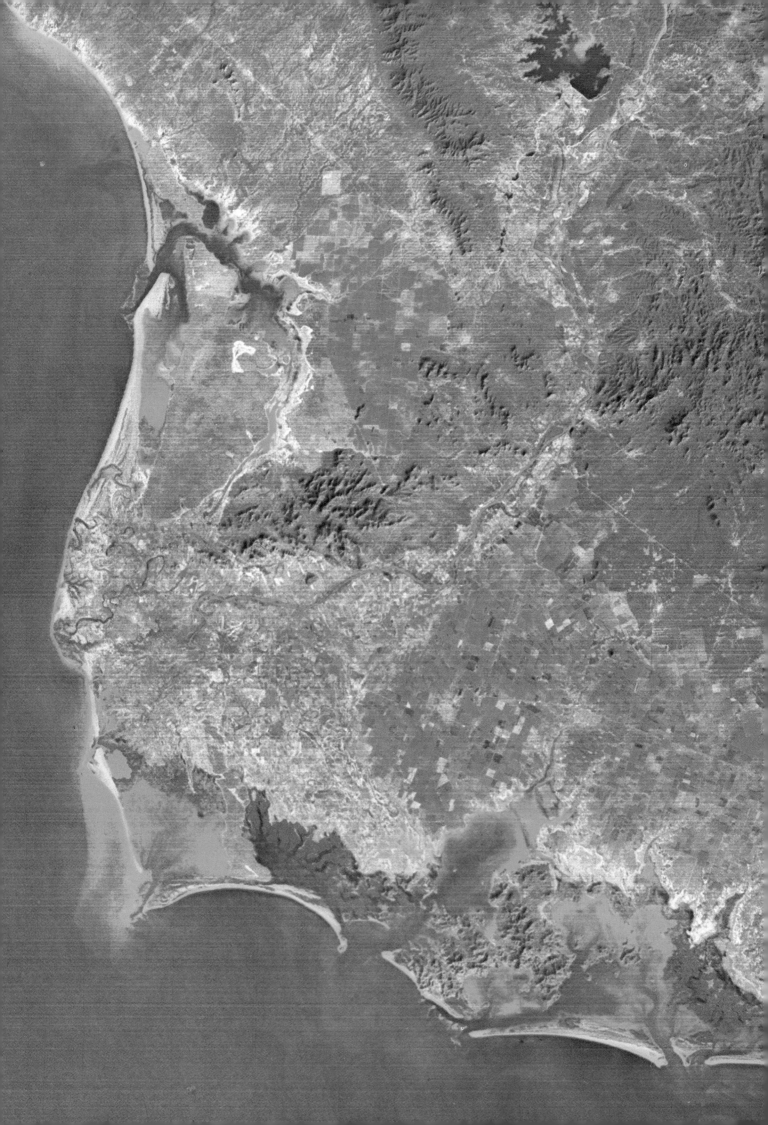

The Agriculture of Mexico

EDWIN J. WELLHAUSEN

The "green revolution" has been a notable success among Mexico's larger, more commercial farmers. Its benefits must now be extended to the majority of rural workers in the traditional farming sectors

Mexico merits a special intermediate position in any comparative international account of agricultural development. In the past 30 years or so Mexico has made remarkable progress in expanding its capacity for producing food, yet many serious problems remain. Having accomplished one agricultural revolution, the country finds itself sorely in need of another. It is this paradox that makes the story of Mexico's agricultural development a particularly instructive case history for inclusion in a review of the state of world agriculture.

The Mexican government has a threefold agricultural policy: (1) to produce enough food and fiber to meet the needs of a growing population; (2) to raise crops that can be exported to bolster foreign exchange; (3) to increase the income and general welfare of the rural people. What has been Mexico's record in recent years in meeting these policy requirements?

During the 1930's and early 1940's food production in Mexico had become stagnant. By 1945 the country was importing between 15 and 20 percent of its cereal grains, mainly corn and wheat, to help supply the food demands of its 22 million people. This situation changed drastically in the next two decades, when there was a striking surge in the production of basic food grains. By 1960 food deficits had disappeared. By 1963 the supply of food began to exceed the domestic demand, and during the next five years considerable quantities of corn and wheat were exported.

Then, in the late 1960's, this dynamic growth began to lose momentum, and by the early 1970's Mexico was again importing between 15 and 20 percent of its basic food grains. Why? What are the problems? What are the prospects for bringing food production back into balance with population growth?

The 20 years from 1950 to 1970 were the boom years in Mexico for food production. In spite of the fact that the population had increased to 43 million by 1965, Mexico managed not only to erase its food deficit but also to generate surpluses for export. According to figures compiled by the National Bank of Mexico, the country exported 5.4 million tons of corn, 1.8 million tons of wheat and 339,000 tons of beans during the period from 1964 to 1969. (Most of the exports were at a loss, since at that time world prices were lower than the government-guaranteed prices.)

Between 1950 and 1970 production of wheat in Mexico increased from 300,000 tons per year to 2.6 million tons—more than eightfold in the short span of 20 years. Yields per unit area quadrupled from 750 kilograms per hectare to 3,200 kilograms. For a time the Mexican government limited the area planted to wheat in order to prevent unmanageable surpluses.

Similarly, but less spectacularly, the output of corn increased by more than 250 percent during the same period: from 3.5 million tons in a good rainfall year in the late 1940's to about nine million in 1968. Average yields per hectare increased from 700 to 1,300 kilograms. Corn is Mexico's staple food crop. Approximately half of the cultivated land is planted to corn every year, most of it under rain-fed conditions.

During the period from 1950 to 1970 the annual bean crop almost doubled: from about 530,000 tons to 925,000.

Corn and beans, eaten in the proportion of about three to one, constitute the main diet of both the rural population and the urban. Much of the protein in the diet is supplied by the beans.

The production of sorghum in 1950 was about 200,000 tons. By 1970 the production of this cereal grain had grown to more than 2.7 million tons per year—a 14-fold increase. In Mexico most of the sorghum crop is used for feeding hogs and poultry. As a result the supply of pork, eggs and chicken increased strikingly to keep pace with the demands of the urban population.

In 1950 soybeans were generally unknown in Mexico, but by 1970 production had increased to some 275,000 tons, adding significantly to the supply of vegetable oils and proteins.

These extraordinary achievements have been referred to in international circles as the "green revolution." Although many economic, political and social factors were involved, the advances were driven largely by a combination of three technological factors: (1) the development of new, high-yielding plant varieties that are widely adaptable, responsive to fertilizer and resistant to disease; (2) the development of an improved "package" of agricultural practices, including better land management, adequate fertilization and more effective control of weeds and insects, all of which made it possible for the improved varieties to more fully realize their high yield potential; (3) a favorable ratio between the cost of fertilizer and other inputs and the price the farmer received for his product.

The first phase of the agricultural revolution in Mexico began in 1943 with the launching of a cooperative agricultural-improvement program by the Mexican Ministry of Agriculture and the Rockefeller Foundation. The stated purpose of the program was to increase the production of the basic food crops through the genetic improvement of plant varieties, the improvement of the soil and the control of insect pests and plant diseases. A corollary goal was to

LARGE-SCALE IRRIGATION has converted the dry northwestern coastal plain of Mexico into one of the country's most productive agricultural regions. The false-color image on the opposite page, made with data obtained on January 11, 1973, by the multispectral scanning system aboard the LANDSAT 1 satellite, shows a portion of this newly fertile strip near the border between the states of Sonora and Sinaloa. The region produces a variety of food crops on a year-round cropping system. Wheat is grown mainly during the cool, dry winter months.

train young men and women in agricultural research and in the development of techniques for promoting the rapid adoption of the new technology. The joint program operated for 16 years (from 1943 to 1959) with a combined multidisciplinary staff in its peak years of 100 Mexican scientists and 20 scientists from other countries. Extraordinary progress was made toward both objectives.

During the quarter of a century from 1945 to 1970 the population of Mexico grew by 220 percent. During the same period corn production increased by 250 percent. Some of this increase resulted from an increase in the area planted to corn, but much of it can be attributed to the increased use of improved seed and chemical fertilizer. Under good conditions some of the improved varieties yielded as much as 100 percent more than the unimproved types.

After extensive experimentation it was found that nitrogen was the principal limiting element in most soils. By the 1950's a hectare of land producing 1,000 kilograms of corn could readily be made to produce at least 4,000 kilograms through the application of 100 kilograms of nitrogen (in the form of various nitrates) in combination with improved seed and adequate moisture. This works out to a ratio of 30 kilograms of corn per kilogram of nitrogen. At that time a kilogram of pure nitrogen cost about four pesos and 30 kilograms of corn was worth 24 pesos. Thus a farmer could realize a sixfold return on money invested in nitrogen (not including other expenses such as the costs of better weed control and of harvesting the additional corn). Before the early 1950's much of the cultivated land was periodically abandoned to grow up in weeds, including wild legumes, because its fertility had diminished to the point where it no longer was economically

feasible to grow a crop on it. That practice was quickly abandoned where money or credit was available to buy chemical fertilizer. This factor alone accounts for much of the increase in land planted to corn and beans during the boom years.

Wheat is grown under irrigation in Mexico during the cool, dry winter months. The wheat varieties available in the 1940's and before then were susceptible to black stem rust, and every year certain fields were completely destroyed or seriously damaged by the pathogen. Because of this hazard farmers did not risk much money, if they risked any, on fertilizer. The situation changed rapidly with the introduction of rust-resistant varieties, which made the application of fertilizer highly profitable. The first rust-resistant varieties were released in the early 1950's, but the big rise in production came in the early 1960's with the release of rust-resistant dwarf varieties. These varieties responded more ef-

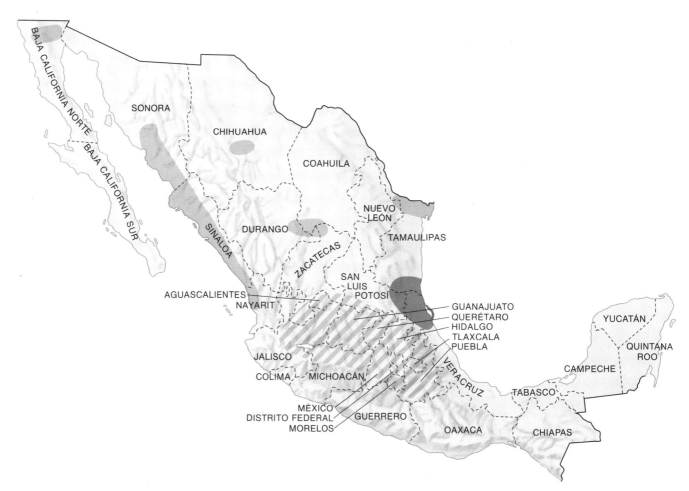

MOUNTAINOUS TOPOGRAPHY OF MEXICO, combined with the very uneven pattern of rainfall, limits the potentially arable land to about 15 percent of the country's total land area. Only about 9 percent of the total is under cultivation today. More than half of the present cropland lies in the predominantly rain-fed central highlands (*hatched area*). Highly productive irrigated areas with varied, year- **round cropping systems include, besides the northwestern coastal plain, portions of the states of Coahuila, Chihuahua, Baja California and Tamaulipas (*light gray areas*). A year-round productive region without irrigation encompasses eastern San Luis Potosí and northern Veracruz (*dark gray area*). Most of the undeveloped potential cropland is in the tropical areas along the coast of the Gulf of Mexico.**

ficiently to greater applications of nitrogen and phosphorus without "lodging" (becoming top-heavy and falling over), and as farmers increased the amounts of fertilizer, unit-area yields began to soar.

Yields of other food crops such as beans, tomatoes, potatoes and sorghum were also greatly increased in those boom years through the application of the new technology. The Food and Agriculture Organization of the United Nations estimated in 1959 that agricultural production in Mexico increased an average of 7 percent per year during the 10-year period ending in 1959. This rate of growth was considerably higher than that achieved by any other country in Latin America.

An important factor in these accomplishments was the intensive in-service training of personnel. Some 750 young men and women participated directly in the field and laboratory phases of the program during the 16 years that it ran. Much of the research work was done in fields in collaboration with the more progressive farmers. The in-service training was not limited to Mexicans; it included people from other Latin-American countries, who were later instrumental in the development of agricultural-improvement programs in their own countries.

In 1952 many of the Mexican trainees entered the production campaign initiated by the Ministry of Agriculture to assist farmers in the application of the new technological package of practices they had helped to develop. Those who demonstrated an aptitude for research and its application in agricultural development were given an opportunity to go abroad and study toward an advanced degree at some of the leading agricultural universities of the world. In 1959 Mexico initiated its own graduate program in agriculture at Chapingo, near Mexico City. Staffed by a well-trained, field-experienced faculty, the school has steadily gained prestige throughout Latin America.

By the late 1960's the impact of this technology-based agricultural revolution appeared to have run its course. Total agricultural production began to level off, and once again the rate of population growth began to exceed the rate of agricultural growth. The increase in the production of corn, for example, first began to level off in 1965 at about nine million tons per year. The demand for corn in 1975, however, reached approximately 10.5 million tons, creating a shortage of about 1.5 million tons. This shortage amounts to about 17 percent, so that in terms of supply and demand the situation has become roughly what it was in 1945. Fortunately supply and demand for other food crops, such as beans, rice, vegetables and sorghum, are approximately in balance. The current deficit is primarily in corn. As a

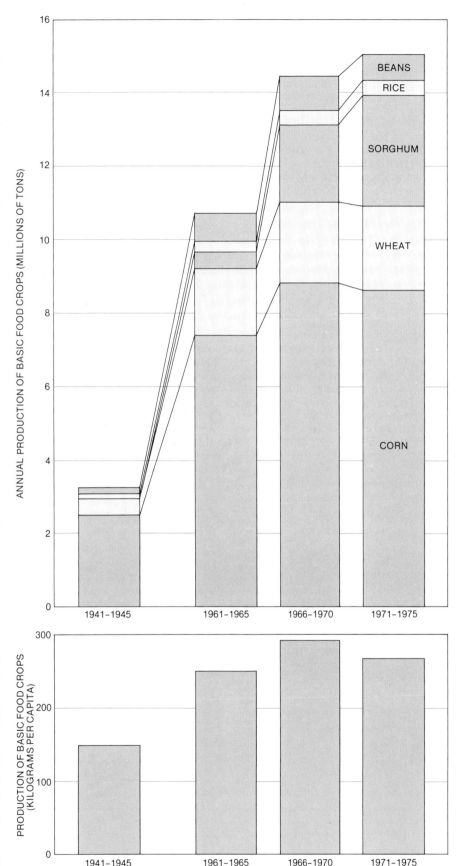

PRODUCTION OF BASIC FOOD CROPS increased dramatically in Mexico in the two decades from 1945 to 1965, after which total food production began to level off as the impact of the technology-based agricultural revolution appeared to have run its course (*bar chart at top*). Since 1970 production per capita has actually declined somewhat (*bar chart at bottom*), as the population (now 62 million) has continued to grow at an annual rate of about 3.5 percent. According to the author, a high rate of growth in agricultural production (in excess of the rate of population growth) can again be achieved in Mexico by promoting the adoption of the recommended "package" of agricultural practices among the large number of comparatively unproductive semicommercial and subsistence farmers in rain-fed areas of the country.

result the importation of cereal grains has risen markedly since 1970.

The current situation can be attributed in part to shifts in government policies regarding cereal production and cost/price ratios, but things appear to be more complicated than that. On careful analysis it is apparent that the production revolution succeeded primarily among the larger, more commercial farmers, who were in a better position to afford the fertilizer and other inputs. Furthermore, as one might expect, the new technologies flourished best in those areas where production risks were the lowest and profit prospects were the highest. All farmers have not benefited equally from the technological advances.

Wheat, for example, is produced largely by the more progressive farmers in the irrigated areas of the Pacific northwest of Mexico and the western part of the central highlands, where water for irrigation is available during the dry winter season; corn, in contrast, has been relegated primarily to the smaller, less advanced farmers in the unirrigated areas, where rainfall is often erratic. New techniques in corn production have been adopted mainly by the more sophisticated commercial farmers in areas where rainfall is generally well distributed during the rainy season. Sor-

ghum, supposedly a crop for dry areas with highly variable rainfall, is being grown mainly by the highly commercial farmers in the better rainfall areas and often under irrigation.

Up to about 1968 the agricultural revolution in Mexico moved ahead mainly under its own momentum without a major effort in technical assistance to the farmers. Could it be that under present circumstances the rate of growth in the production of food crops has diminished because the rural sector is running out of clients who can make use of the technological package in the form in which it is now being offered? Is there a need to develop special technological packages better suited to unirrigated areas where rainfall is often poorly distributed? Must the programs of technical assistance be reoriented at the farmer level to gain more rapid adoption of profitable technology by a larger proportion of farmers? Is the current deficit likely to become chronic because Mexico is running out of arable land? These questions call for a closer examination of the present character and the future problems of Mexico's agriculture.

The total land area of Mexico is some 195 million hectares—roughly a fourth the area of the U.S. According to existing estimates, about 30 million hec-

tares, or 15 percent of the total area, is potentially arable, but only about 16,-776,000 hectares, or 8.6 percent, is under cultivation today. This is only a little more than the total area of cultivated land in the state of Iowa. The rest of the land is either too dry, too wet or too mountainous for the raising of crops. Most of the undeveloped potential cropland is in the low-lying tropical areas. Much of it is poorly drained, permanently flooded or periodically inundated and is subject to hazards that make it an unsatisfactory place for people to live. The investment needed to bring it into cultivation would be very large.

More than half of the present cropland lies in the rain-fed central highlands. In this region annual rainfall varies widely, most of it coming in a period of four months, from July through October. Moreover, the rainfall is often irregular during the rainy season. Although most of the crops are grown under rain-fed conditions, supplemental irrigation is available for about 1.5 million hectares. The main crop in the area is corn, but other crops such as wheat, vegetables (tomatoes in particular), strawberries and potatoes are grown during the winter months where irrigation is available. The central highlands constitute only about 15 percent of the total area of Mexico, but they include

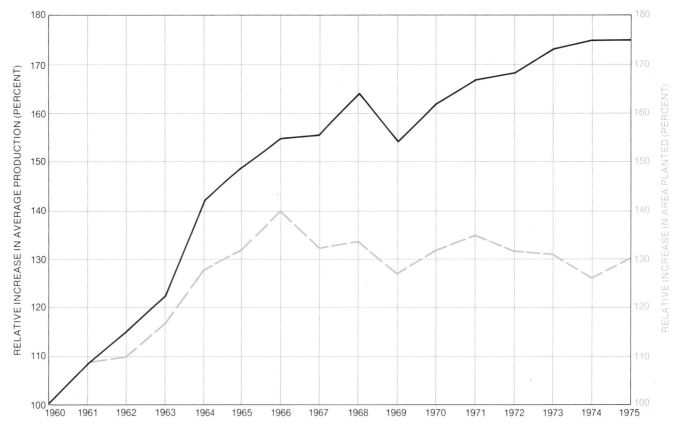

RECENT LEVELING TREND in the aggregate output of Mexico's 25 leading crops is evident in this graph, which summarizes the data for the past 15 years according to two different indexes of agricultural growth: the average annual production (*black curve*) and the total area planted (*colored curve*). The 25 crops are corn, wheat, rice, sorghum, barley, beans, soybeans, potatoes, tomatoes, onions, garlic, chick-peas, alfalfa, strawberries, melons, watermelons, sugar, cotton, coffee, cacao, tobacco, sesame, peanuts, flax and safflower.

not only half of the country's total cropland but also more than half of the total population.

One of the most productive agricultural areas in Mexico is in the dry northwestern coastal plain under irrigation in the states of Sonora and Sinaloa. This region produces considerable quantities of wheat, vegetables, rice, soybeans, sugarcane, cotton, safflower and sorghum in a year-round cropping system. Here yields per unit area are among the highest in the world.

Smaller but still highly productive irrigated areas with similar cropping patterns are located in the states of Coahuila, Chihuahua, Baja California and Tamaulipas. Another year-round productive area encompasses eastern San Luis Potosí and northern Veracruz, where the rainfall is fairly well distributed throughout the year. Although this area is unirrigated, it produces considerable quantities of corn, sugarcane and tropical fruits.

With few exceptions, the remaining land currently cultivated is widely dispersed on steep slopes, narrow ridges and small alluvial valley floors throughout the eastern and western mountain ranges and southern highlands. In these areas traditional semicommercial and subsistence agriculture involving corn and beans prevails. In the eastern mountains and southern highlands, with the exception of some of the highland valleys in Oaxaca, rainfall is usually adequate during six months of the year.

According to an analysis made by the National Bank of Mexico, there are 2,816,000 farm units in Mexico. Of these, 7.1 percent are classified as modern, consisting of those farms on which the more progressive, commercially minded farmers apply the recommended package of improved technological practices more or less completely; 40.5 percent are classified as traditional semicommercial farms, on many of which the farmers apply at least part of the recommended agricultural practices, and 52.4 percent are classified as subsistence farms, cultivated by farmers who buy or sell very little and are mainly concerned with producing enough corn and beans for themselves and their families. As one might expect, there are striking differences in the average farm size, percent of cropland under irrigation, capital investment and average gross income among the three categories. The rapid increase of agricultural production during the boom years is due primarily to the efforts of the modern sector.

About 50 percent of the total farm units are located in the central highlands. In this region landholdings average 10.7 hectares per unit, of which about six hectares is suitable for raising crops. It is in this area that the problems of overcrowding and subsistence agri-

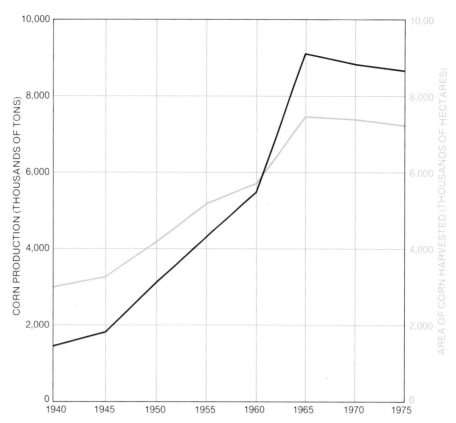

ANNUAL PRODUCTION OF CORN in Mexico grew at a rate faster than the rate of population increase between 1945 and 1965, when the crop began to flatten out at a level of about nine million tons per year (*black curve*). Some of the increase during the boom years resulted from an increase in the area planted to corn (*colored curve*), but much of it can be attributed to increased yield. Close to 98 percent of the corn crop is consumed in the form of tortillas.

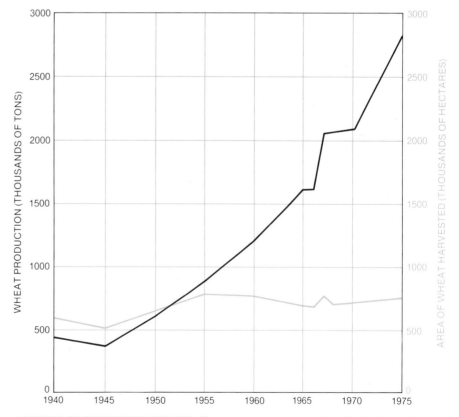

ANNUAL PRODUCTION OF WHEAT grew even more spectacularly during the peak years for Mexican agriculture, with yields per unit area quadrupling between 1950 and 1970. The extremely high yields obtained in recent years under irrigated conditions with the new disease-resistant dwarf varieties of wheat are reflected in this graph, which compares the annual output of wheat (*black curve*) with the number of hectares harvested each year (*colored curve*).

culture are severest. Many of the subsistence farms are located in marginal areas of poor soil and inadequate rainfall.

In the country as a whole a comparatively small number of modern farmers provide about 45 percent of the total commercial agricultural production on about 20 percent of the cropland. In contrast, the large semicommercial and subsistence sectors combined account for about 55 percent of the total agricultural production on about 80 percent of the total cropland. Farmers in the latter group operate primarily under rain-fed conditions, and their production has generally become stagnant. In many places rainfall is often insufficient and variable, yet it is estimated that about three-fourths of the farmers in the semicommercial and subsistence sectors are economically viable and could profitably and substantially increase their production through the application of modern technology.

The third of the total cropland in Mexico that is irrigated provides about 55 percent of the total agricultural production. Although much more supplemental irrigation could be provided in many of the rain-fed areas, the development of additional full-scale irrigation projects in present agricultural areas does not seem promising. Practically all the water sources on the surface and underground are already being utilized. Putting additional land under full-scale irrigation would be extremely costly. In some of the irrigated regions of the central highlands water shortages are becoming increasingly apparent and groundwater tables are falling.

Irrigated areas not only are more productive but also have a tremendous advantage in that they can produce a wide range of crops in multiple-cropping systems, including fruits and vegetables with high net returns. Rain-fed agriculture is limited to corn, beans, sorghum and chick-peas.

The present population of Mexico is about 62 million, with an annual rate of growth of about 3.5 percent. (The comparatively high growth rate of the population is a reflection not only of a high fertility rate but also of a rapidly falling death rate.) Some 40 percent of the total population, or about 23 million, live or work in the rural areas. Of these, 5.1 million are classified as being economically active, with 3.5 million of them considered to be underemployed. If the present population growth rate continues, the rural population can be expected to increase greatly and along with it the number of underemployed, many of whom will seek work in the cities. The present industrial and service sectors can in no way provide employment for the growing numbers of rural unemployed or underemployed.

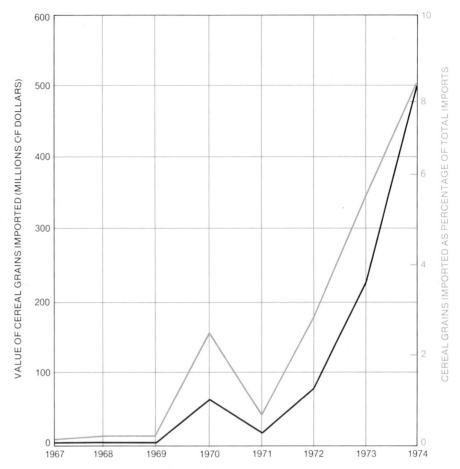

IMPORTATION OF CEREAL GRAINS into Mexico has increased sharply in recent years, owing to the growing deficit in corn production. The required level of grain imports is plotted here in terms of dollar value (*black curve*) and percentage of total imports (*colored curve*).

Although a great effort is being made to improve rural education, the educational levels of the farming groups in the semicommercial and subsistence categories continue to be very low. It will be easier to convert the subsistence population in marginally productive regions into a reasonably productive agricultural labor force than to try to incorporate them into the industrial world. It is essential that the agricultural sector itself provide greater opportunities for employment.

Mexico has millions of hectares of good, reasonably level, potentially fertile cropland in the north-central plateau and in the northwestern coastal plains. These regions could produce millions of tons of additional food crops—if enough water were available. In these areas crop production is not possible without irrigation, and most of the available water is already being utilized.

One of the basic problems of Mexican agriculture is that the distribution of the water resources does not coincide with the distribution of the good cropland. The currently cropped land and the people are concentrated in the drier or semiarid areas of the country. The central highlands, for example, which have about half of the population and half of

the cropland, have only about 10 percent of the water resources. In contrast, the southeastern region, which has only 8 percent of the population and very little cropland, has 40 percent of the water resources. The available water is obviously not where it is needed most or where it can best be utilized.

The crops Mexico produces for export are primarily cotton, sugarcane, strawberries, tomatoes, onions, melons and watermelons. With the exception of sugarcane these crops are grown mostly under irrigated conditions during the dry season of the year. Up to 1973 the agricultural sector generated more than half of Mexico's total income from exports. A combination of factors caused this proportion to drop to about 33 percent in 1974. A reduction in cotton exports had its effect, but it is becoming increasingly clear that the general stagnation in the production of the basic food crops was a major factor in the decline.

Some four million tons of grain (mostly corn, but including wheat and sorghum) were imported for the 1974–1975 consumption year. This large volume of imports was needed in part because of the vagaries of the weather and the almost complete exhaustion of reserves. An increase in prices on the world market raised the costs of these imports by 103 percent over previous years. At the same time prices on Mexican export products increased by only 20 percent. In view of this situation the Mexican government is again making a strong effort to accelerate the production of basic food crops, even at the expense of export crops. Imports for the 1975–1976 consumption year are calculated to be about 1.7 million tons, again mostly corn.

Price manipulations are a powerful tool for increasing or limiting the production of certain crops in Mexico. In order to stimulate the production of basic food crops and to promote self-sufficiency, guaranteed prices were sharply increased in 1974. This policy represents a striking change from the period between 1968 and 1972, when average prices increased at an annual rate of only 3 percent. Guaranteed prices for corn, wheat and sorghum were further increased in 1975.

Although most farmers do not receive the government-guaranteed prices, the prices they do receive are influenced by them and have risen sharply. The costs of inputs have also greatly increased but not nearly as much as the market price of the grain. The cost of fertilizer, one of the main ingredients in the recommended package of practices, has increased only 12 percent. Today the ratio of input costs to product price in the basic food crops is extremely favorable. At current prices it takes only three kilograms of corn or wheat to pay for one kilogram of nitrogen. Each kilogram of nitrogen applied, costing about four and a half pesos, will conservatively yield an average of 10 kilograms of grain worth 15 pesos. Under irrigation or in rain-fed areas where rainfall is well distributed a kilogram of nitrogen will produce up to 30 kilograms of grain. Food-crop production today can be very profitable, even with significant increases in the costs of labor, fuel, agricultural machinery and transportation.

The consumption of fertilizer in Mexico grew at the rate of 12 percent per year in the 1960's. During that decade the use of nitrogen more than tripled: from 118,000 tons in 1960 to 380,000 tons in 1970. Similarly, the use of phosphorus (in the form of phosphates) grew from 43,000 tons in 1960 to 115,000 tons in 1970—an increase of 270 percent. This sharp upward trend has continued: in 1974, 551,000 tons of nitrogen and 183,000 tons of phosphorus were used. Since Mexico is self-sufficient in petroleum, most of the nitrogen is now locally produced.

Crop research played a significant role in the rapid acceleration of grain production in the first phase of the Mexican agricultural revolution. Nicolás Ardito Barletti, a Panamanian, attempted to place a value on the social benefit from research and its applications during the boom years. According to his estimate, the investment made in all research from 1945 on was paying dividends by 1965 at the rate of 300 percent per year. Investments in wheat research alone paid dividends at the rate of 700 percent per year. Although these high returns were in part due to the fact that the agricultural conditions subject to improvement in 1945, when it all started, were primitive even in the more dynamic sector, it is clear that research played a key role in triggering the returns.

Responsibility for agricultural research today rests with the National Institute of Agricultural Research, created in 1960. The institute, with its headquarters at Chapingo, now operates eight regional research stations located in different parts of the country. All the stations are well equipped physically, but unfortunately, with the supply and demand of basic food crops in balance and with the surplus problems in the 1960's, the pressure was off and many of the stations began to become less active. Owing to low salaries and the lack of career opportunities, Mexico's most competent agricultural research workers began to become widely dispersed in administrative positions and other more remunerative activities and were replaced by younger and less experienced people. With the leaders gone, these young workers, although highly capable, were handicapped by the lack of the guidance and leadership formerly supplied by the more experienced researchers. As a result research has in many areas tended to become stagnant (except in the case of wheat research, which is supported in large part by the International Maize and Wheat Improvement Center). The lack of a dynamic on-farm research program and the lack of an adequate farmer-education system have been the primary factors in preventing the spread of modern technology to a greater number of farmers.

In recent years technical education has been expanded. Mexico now has seven agricultural schools at the undergraduate level, two of which are giving graduate training leading to an M.S. degree. In 1974, 188 students were awarded advanced degrees in botany, entomology, plant pathology, genetics, soil improvement, irrigation, agricultural economics and rural development. This is a good beginning, but many more people with a fundamental knowledge of the basic sciences and rural-development skills will be needed.

In an attempt to stimulate agricultural production, allocations of public funds to the agricultural sector have increased more than 700 percent in Mexico since 1970. In terms of 1970 dollars this represents an increase from $443 million in 1970 to $3.2 billion in 1975; in terms of total government expenditures it represents an increase from 7.6 percent to 20.1 percent.

Of these increases the Ministry of Hydraulic Resources received $568 million, or about 18 percent, three-fourths of which was to be spent on expanding irrigation works. Budgets for research and for promoting a more rapid adoption of research results were also substantially increased. A separate agency

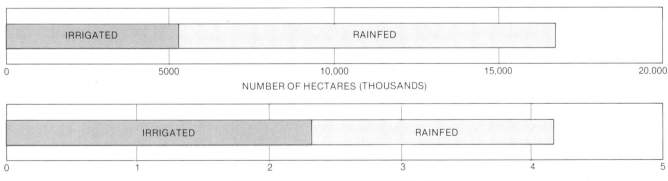

IRRIGATED CROPLAND generates more than half of the total commercial output of Mexico's farms, measured in dollars (*lower bar*), even though the area under irrigation comprises only about 30 percent of the total cropland, measured in hectares (*upper bar*). The irrigated regions, in addition to their superior productivity, can yield a wider range of crops on the basis of multiple-cropping systems.

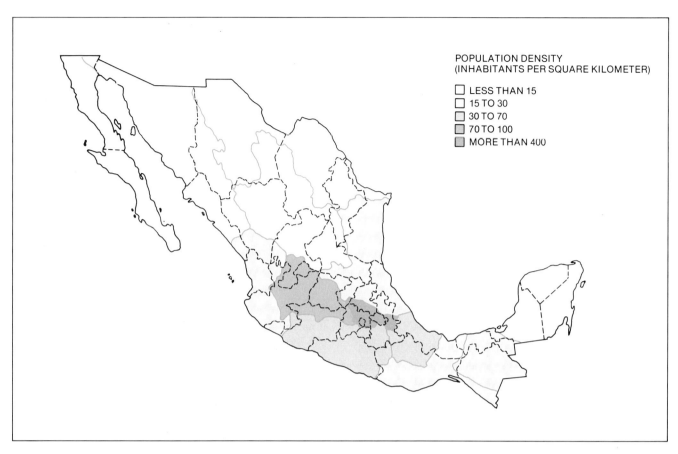

POPULATION DENSITY
(INHABITANTS PER SQUARE KILOMETER)

☐ LESS THAN 15
☐ 15 TO 30
☐ 30 TO 70
◫ 70 TO 100
▩ MORE THAN 400

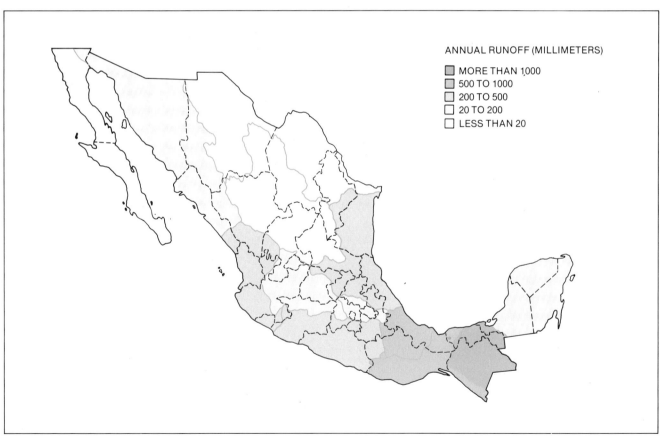

ANNUAL RUNOFF (MILLIMETERS)

▩ MORE THAN 1,000
◫ 500 TO 1000
☐ 200 TO 500
☐ 20 TO 200
☐ LESS THAN 20

A BASIC PROBLEM confronting agricultural planners in Mexico is that the distribution of the population (*map at top*) does not coincide with the distribution of the water resources (*map at bottom*). Thus most of the people (and most of the farms) are concentrated in the drier areas of the country, particularly in the central highlands, which have more than half of the population but only about 10 percent of the water resources. In contrast, approximately 40 percent of the country's available water supply is in the humid southeastern region, where only about 8 percent of the people live. The two maps on this page are based on data obtained by the Mexican Ministry of Hydraulic Resources; for comparative statistical purposes the country is divided on both of the maps into 13 major hydrologic regions.

for agricultural extension was organized in 1970 and since then has grown in budget and personnel at an annual rate of 49 percent. In 1970 technical assistance was provided for 604,000 hectares of farmland. By 1974 that figure had risen to 2.9 million hectares. The number of technical-assistance agents increased at an annual rate of 42 percent to a total of 3,352 in 1975. So far the payoff from these increased investments in technical assistance has been disappointing, however, owing largely to the lack of skilled personnel.

The foregoing analysis of the current state of agriculture in Mexico will have set in the foreground a number of facts bearing on the further acceleration of food production in Mexico. First, there is the dual nature of Mexico's agriculture: on the one hand a small, progressive modern sector providing the major portion of the commercial agricultural products and on the other a large, comparatively unproductive semicommercial and subsistence farming sector concerned primarily with providing enough food for the farmers and their families to eat. Second, there is the problem of the limited and irregular supply of water for crop production in the principal agricultural areas. Third, on the positive side, there is the strenuous effort on the part of government officials to stimulate a new surge in food production.

The job ahead is a formidable one. If grain production is to be brought into balance with demand, the annual rate of increase during the next decade must be about 5 percent. Although the modern sector, with more than 70 percent of the present irrigation facilities, can produce still more through more intensive cropping systems and a more efficient use of seasonal rains and irrigation water, the greatest immediate potential for increasing food production is in the large traditional farming sector in areas with a high annual rainfall. This sector at present is producing only a fraction of what it could with the widespread application of modern technology.

In spite of the fact that more beans, rice and sorghum will also be needed, the major concern continues to be corn; the degree to which Mexico will maintain its self-sufficiency in food production will depend primarily on the rate at which the production of this crop is increased. According to the best estimates that can be made from the available statistics, the area annually planted to corn today varies between six and eight million hectares. Of this area roughly 620,000 hectares, or about 10 percent, is grown under irrigation or with some supplemental irrigation. The rest is planted under rain-fed conditions, mostly by the semicommercial farmers.

On the basis of estimates made by the National Institute of Agricultural Research one can compare the amount of corn currently being raised on deep and shallow soils in five different rainfall regimes with what could be produced in each of these regimes with the aid of modern technology [*see illustration on pages 96 and 97*]. From such studies it appears that the application of the technological package in its present form is not economically feasible in regimes with an annual rainfall of less than 700 millimeters and a drought probability of more than 35 percent. The main potential for increased corn production, therefore, is limited to the more humid areas.

It is evident from such data that the present annual production of 6,739,000 tons of corn in the areas of higher rainfall could be increased to more than 25 million tons—almost quadrupled—with the more complete exploitation of available technology. This possibility is exciting, and if it is realized, it could not only keep Mexico self-sufficient in corn for the next two decades but also provide a substantial increase in income for a large proportion of the semicommercial and subsistence farmers. In these areas, at the present cost/price ratio, farmers can expect a return of 100 percent on investments in fertilizer in good years. It is possible that the present technological package, with certain modifications, could even be extended to some of the areas of less rainfall and thus further increase the projected potential for corn.

The substantial increase in the number of hectares in the projections for the more humid areas is based on the assumption that the present custom of periodically abandoning good cropland for fertility restoration will completely disappear with the widespread applica-

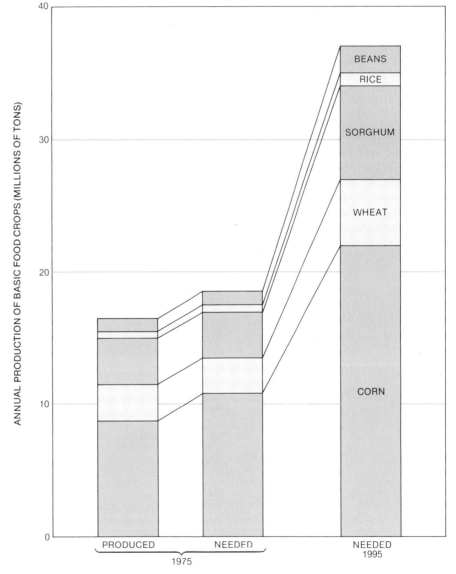

DIMENSIONS OF THE TASK AHEAD if Mexico is to avoid large imports of food in the future are suggested by these three bars, which compare the amount of five basic food crops produced and needed in Mexico in 1975 with the amount that will be needed by 1995 if the present rate of population growth continues. According to the author, the country has enough cropland and water resources to meet its own food requirements for the next three decades.

tion of chemical fertilizer. Since beans are generally planted in association with corn, it is possible that the additional supplies of this crop needed by 1995 could also be produced in the higher-rainfall areas with the aid of improved technology.

In the realization of this enormous potential many obstacles must be overcome. More practical on-farm research will be needed to determine the precise fertilizer requirements and agronomic practices most economic for each of the different ecological situations in which corn and beans can be efficiently grown. This task must be combined with studies in the fields of agricultural economics and the social sciences in order to better understand the problems and motivations of the traditional farmer. Furthermore, new strategies for gaining rapid adoption of new production technology by large numbers of poorly motivated semicommercial and subsistence farmers will need to be worked out for each community. Conventional systems that have been so effective in the diffusion of modern technology among the more sophisticated farmers are of little value in the more conservative semicommercial and subsistence sectors.

These farmers will need more direct assistance in the commercialization of their operations. Their motivations and problems must be more clearly understood. Their fear of change must be alleviated. New incentives for change must

be created and encouraged. More adequate systems of facilitating credit will need to be developed. Many problems in the distribution of material inputs must be solved, and better marketing and storage facilities must be provided.

It is not likely that the obstacles will be overcome without the development of a new cadre of well-supported, production-minded, rural-improvement agents who understand the problems to be solved and are experienced in the strategies to be followed. Such agents will have to be willing to work at close range with the small farmer in increasing his production and income and in helping him to create a better life for himself and his family where he is, so that he is not obliged to seek new opportunities in the already overcrowded cities. Once the new agents are at work in the field and a strong desire to produce more and live better is instilled in the traditional farming sector, the demand for credit, material, inputs and better facilities for marketing and storage will soon iron out the many difficulties now encountered in the efficient provision of these things.

Thanks to the vision of a small group of workers in the graduate school at Chapingo and in the nearby International Maize and Wheat Improvement Center, a pilot program for the development, testing and application of strategies for accelerating the production of corn and the socioeconomic progress of the semicommercial and subsistence

farmer was established in a rain-fed area in the state of Puebla in 1967. This highly successful project has clearly identified the many problems and constraints facing the local farmer and has demonstrated a number of effective strategies for their solution. The success of this research project will undoubtedly be an important factor in accelerating the large rural-development investment program recently initiated by the government of Mexico.

The Puebla project has demonstrated that small farmers operating under rain-fed conditions can profitably exploit modern technology. Even when the more productive techniques are successfully demonstrated, however, the risk of losses from drought, hail, unseasonal frosts and floods appears to be a major constraint in their widespread adoption. To compensate small farmers for such losses the government has provided an effective insurance program, the coverage of which was increased from 1.9 million hectares in 1973 to 2.6 million in 1974, a gain of 36 percent in one year.

The further development of supplemental irrigation in the form of tube wells, another solution being investigated by the Ministry of Hydraulic Resources, would have an even greater effect in promoting the quicker adoption of the new technology under rain-fed conditions. The potential gains from this approach seem to be much greater than those from the development of additional full-scale irrigation projects.

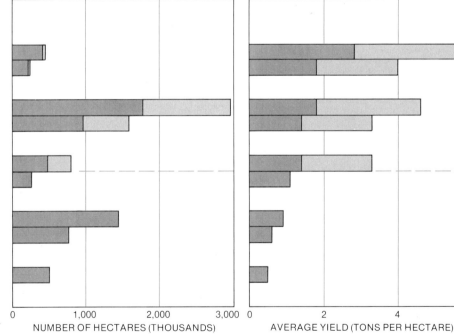

RAINFALL REGIME	DROUGHT PROBABILITY (PERCENT)	SOIL
IRRIGATED	0	DEEP
		SHALLOW
800 TO 900 MILLIMETERS	20	DEEP
		SHALLOW
700 TO 800 MILLIMETERS	35	DEEP
		SHALLOW
600 TO 700 MILIMETERS	45	DEEP
		SHALLOW
<600 MILLIMETERS	60	—

NUMBER OF HECTARES (THOUSANDS)   AVERAGE YIELD (TONS PER HECTARE)

POTENTIAL for increased corn production in Mexico is represented by the colored increments associated with each bar in this chart, which compares the amount of corn currently being raised on deep and shallow soils in five different rainfall regimes with what could be produced in each of these regimes with the aid of modern technology. The chart is based on estimates made by the National Institute of Agricultural Research near Mexico City. The general conclusion drawn from such statistics is that the application of the recommended package of agricultural practices would be economically feasible for farmers in areas with an annual rainfall of more than 700 mil-

Where supplemental irrigation is feasible the risks of low yields or crop failure due to drought could be eliminated. In such areas supplemental irrigation not only would ensure the farmer a substantial return on his investment in fertilizer, good seed, insecticides and additional labor but also would add a substantial quantity of grain to the national breadbasket. With the diffusion of modern technology in the Puebla project the demand for tube wells has greatly increased, and many new communally operated wells have been established.

Supplemental irrigation would remove many of the risks of dry years in the more humid areas. Moreover, it could extend modern production techniques into certain areas with less rainfall. Unless this can be done it is not likely that the nearly three million hectares now being planted annually to corn in the marginal low-rainfall areas will contribute much to increasing the commercial production of this crop, at least in the near future. There are those who maintain that this vast area might gradually be freed for the production of other crops such as sorghum, millet and pasture for livestock, which are generally considered to be more efficient under low and erratic rainfall conditions. The fact remains that corn is the main subsistence crop for the people living in these areas, and they are not likely to substitute anything else for the corn in their diet. Although the present package of technology is not economically feasible for them, new packages based on the planting of improved high-yielding, early-maturing, drought-tolerant varieties of corn, in combination with small quantities of chemical fertilizer and moisture-preserving techniques, could be developed; such techniques might be highly profitable over a period of, say, 10 years. This possibility is practically untouched by research workers today.

Concurrently with special efforts at increasing corn production under rain-fed conditions, research on ways of making the full-scale irrigation projects still more productive must be intensified. In frost-free areas it should be possible to grow three or four crops annually where only two are now being grown. In areas susceptible to frost wheat is an excellent crop for winter production. At present wheat yields average about 3,600 kilograms per hectare. Yields could be readily increased to 6,000 or 7,000 kilograms. Some farmers are already producing 6,000 kilograms per hectare, and at the experimental stations yields as high as 10,000 kilograms are being obtained with the new varieties.

Studies are now being made to evaluate the construction of water-control systems for the very rainy tropical lowland areas of southeastern Mexico. With the proper preparation 150,000 hectares of new land could be brought into year-round crop production almost immediately. During the next decade three million additional hectares could be added. Although this effort would be very costly, it would open up tremendous new food-production possibilities. Rice production, for example, could be shifted from the dry irrigated Pacific coastal plains to the humid Gulf coast lowlands. Similarly, sugarcane, which is also adapted to humid conditions, could be shifted from the Pacific northwest to the southeast, thereby freeing thousands of hectares for the labor-intensive production of food crops more easily handled in dry climates. With water control corn would also be an excellent crop in the southeast during the rainy season.

To make this possibility a reality would require extensive research in cropping systems and soil management. Under high rainfall conditions good land, once its natural vegetation is removed, loses its productivity rapidly without special cropping and management systems. In exploring this possibility the experiences of the International Institute of Tropical Agriculture in the rain forests of Nigeria and those of tropical research institutes in other areas would be very helpful to Mexico's agricultural research workers.

At the present rate of population growth Mexico will need to increase its basic grain production from 16 million tons per year to 37 million by 1995 if large imports are to be avoided. Government officials have a strong desire to do so, and the country has enough cropland and water resources that could be more efficiently exploited in making this goal a reality. Thus Mexico is in an excellent position to meet its own food requirements for the next three decades. The development of this potential not only will greatly increase Mexico's food supplies but also could provide many new opportunities for more remunerative employment of people who are currently underemployed.

Many of the essentials for Mexico's second agricultural revolution are in place. All the key positions in the Ministry of Agriculture are filled with capable, enthusiastic officials who gained considerable practical experience in the field during the earlier boom period. All are academically well trained in the basic agricultural sciences. Many other experienced, well-trained workers who participated in the first production revolution are now teaching in the graduate school at Chapingo and in some of the other leading agricultural schools throughout the country. So far government officials have substantially increased national fertilizer production capacities; they have established pricing policies extremely favorable to the application of modern production techniques, and they have sharply increased the funds available for general agricultural development.

Increasing the production of the traditional sector under rain-fed conditions will be much more difficult than increasing the production of the modern sector during the boom years. To accomplish this task will require (1) a more precise definition of highly profitable technological production techniques for each of the many different ecological regions; (2) more effective strategies for gaining widespread adoption of the techniques; (3) a large, experienced multidisciplinary team of experts who are willing to work in close association with the farmers, teaching them and encouraging them to new levels of productivity.

If the modern sector is to double its production in the next two decades, more intensive cropping patterns will have to be developed and yields of all crops will have to be increased. All of this will require more sophisticated research. Production increases in the southeast will not come merely through water control. Agricultural scientists must learn how to make the new croplands increasingly more productive in spite of torrential rains and hurricane winds. They must then teach the new techniques to the farmers on whom the increases in food production will in the final analysis depend.

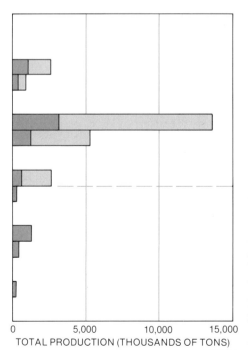

0   5,000   10,000   15,000
TOTAL PRODUCTION (THOUSANDS OF TONS)

limeters and a drought probability of less than 35 percent; this threshold is indicated by broken colored line across middle of chart. Corn production could in that case be roughly tripled, to more than 27 million tons.

9

The Agriculture of India

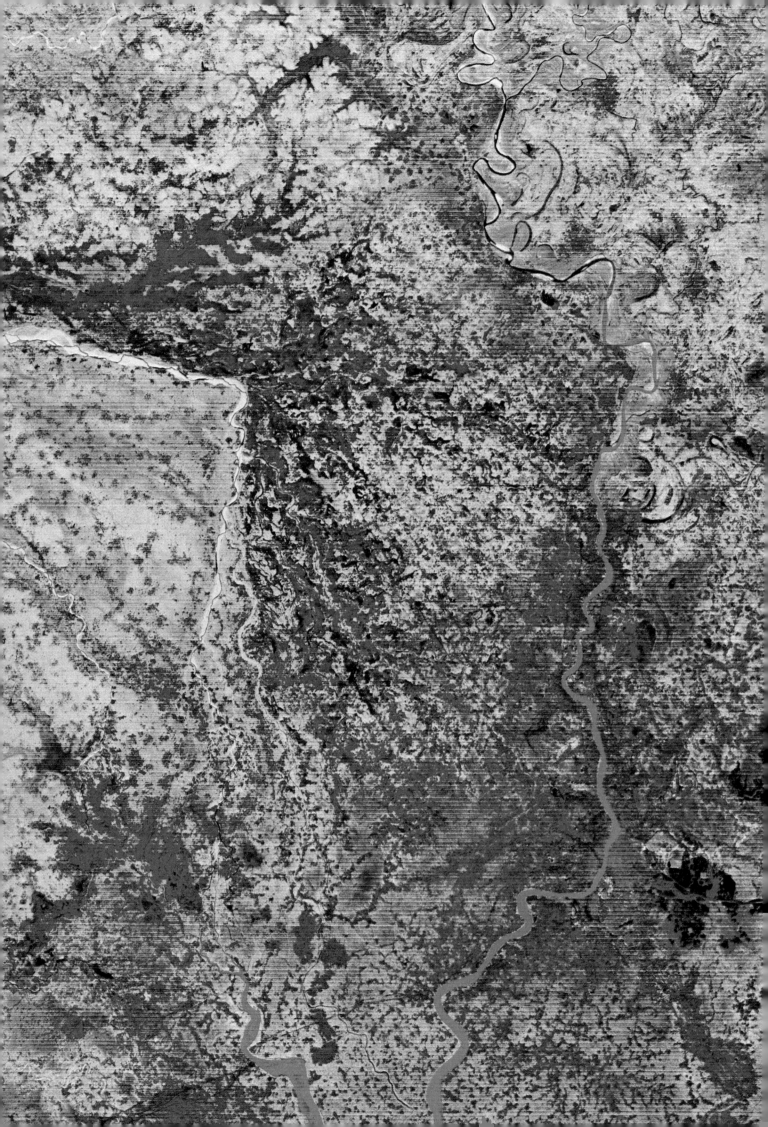

The Agriculture of India

JOHN W. MELLOR

The nation has done much better in feeding its great population than most outsiders realize. Increasing farm output still more may force hard choices among strategies of agricultural and industrial growth.

Contrary to standard stereotypes, India increased its production of food grains approximately 2.8 percent per year from 1950 to the present, a rate significantly higher than the population growth rate of about 2.1 percent for the same period. The result has been a modest improvement in diets and a substantial decline in death rates. That is in sharp contrast to the last several decades of the colonial period, prior to 1947, when food-grain production virtually stagnated, with an insignificant .11 percent per year growth rate, as population was growing at a rate of 1.5 percent per year. In the last decades of colonialism India's capacity to feed itself deteriorated rapidly as a consequence of an effort to provide the exportable surpluses expected of a colony. The result was not only a growing food and welfare problem but also a legacy of poverty and institutions inappropriate for development. Both would impede growth for decades.

Compared with China, the other huge low-income country, India has achieved a somewhat higher rate of increase in food-grain production, albeit a rate of increase from a substantially lower base of average yields and lower proportion of land area irrigated. Making precise comparisons between the two countries is difficult, given differences in the years when production was depressed by weather or internal disturbances and differences in reporting systems. Subject to such complexities, the long-term growth trend in Chinese grain produc-

tion in the period since 1950 is estimated at 2 percent per year, compared with the 2.8 percent for India.

India has a population of 600 million (two-thirds that of China and nearly three times that of the U.S.), is the fourth-largest grain producer in the world and has one of the largest potentials of any nation for future increases in grain production. Given India's central place in the world food situation, it is crucial that close analysis of past trends, of the nature of the future potentials and of the essentials of appropriate investment and political policy be substituted for the existing stereotypes of the Indian food economy. The bases of these stereotypes are four, and in themselves they explain much of the nature of India's food problems and food requirements.

First, India experiences substantial year-to-year fluctuations in its weather and in the past has had a tendency to fill the resulting gaps in food supplies by imports rather than by the more costly domestic storage. Thus in the postindependence period, although there have been substantial year-to-year fluctuations in grain imports, there has been no upward or downward trend in their relative importance. China's record in this respect has been surprisingly similar, including the scale of the imports and the emphasis on supplying the major urban centers.

Second, India, unlike China, maintained its ties with the developed nations

and therefore substantially employed food-aid channels rather than commercial ones for its imports, which tended to overpublicize the periodic domestic shortfalls. Third, and perhaps most important, since India did not have a massive sociopolitical revolution comparable to China's, it has a distribution of income essentially the same as that of the U.S. The result is that in a country as poor on the average as postcolonial India is, there is a large proportion of people who even in normal times do not have enough income to get food through market processes and who in times of crop failure are subject to extreme stress and even famine. The Indian system of government, unlike the Chinese, is not suited to acquiring sufficient control of production through coercive measures to alleviate such stress.

Fourth, agricultural development is largely a process of institutional change that is necessarily slow. The myth of India's relatively poor food performance impedes analysis of the extent to which such changes are occurring and hence analysis of the basis for future growth. In addition there is a reduced rationale for analysis of the extraordinarily rich Indian experience in agricultural development, from the Community Development Program to the Intensive Agricultural District Program and the Small and Marginal Farmers Program. All three not only offer important lessons for the solution of the world food problem but also have led to an evolution of mature domestic institutions servicing the agricultural sector that is generally not comprehended by the now less involved Western advisers of developing countries.

In a country such as India agriculture is central to the economy. Nearly half of the country's gross national product is generated in agriculture; more than half of all consumer expenditures are for food. In years of poor crops total consumer expenditures consistently decline, and there is an even greater decrease in industrial investment. It is now

FINE-GRAINED TEXTURE of landholdings typical of Indian agriculture is evident in this false-color LANDSAT view of the state of West Bengal, where in the opinion of many agronomists agricultural productivity has been hampered by a system of petty landlords, each of whom typically owns about four hectares of cropland, which is in turn worked by three or four tenant farmers and their families. The overall scale of this scene, recorded by LANDSAT 2 from an altitude of some 570 miles on March 29, 1975, is the same as that of the scenes of American and Mexican agricultural patterns reproduced on pages 2, 76, and 86. Notwithstanding the comparatively poor performance of the fertile eastern Gangetic Plain at present, the region is richly endowed with groundwater and is considered to have a great potential for agricultural growth. Light blue area at lower right is Calcutta, the capital of West Bengal. The large river flowing through city is the Hooghly, the westernmost channel of the Ganges Delta.

well established that people with low incomes will spend the bulk of any increased income on food. The lesson is clear: a strategy of growth that mobilizes low-income people for production purposes will give rise to a greater drain on the food supply than would be the case if they were left unemployed or marginally employed.

On the other hand, a strategy that stresses the growth of capital-intensive heavy industry at the expense of agriculture and the less capital-intensive consumer goods combines a static farm output with a slower increase in the demand for food, since capital-intensive industrialization yields its income benefits to a smaller fraction of the population. Thus agricultural policy involves much more than a race between food and population: it fundamentally determines

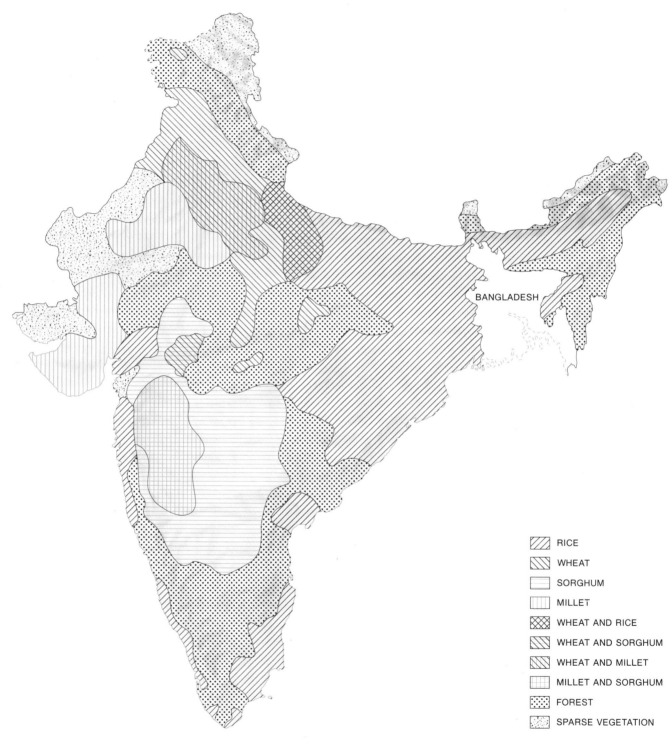

RICE

WHEAT

SORGHUM

MILLET

WHEAT AND RICE

WHEAT AND SORGHUM

WHEAT AND MILLET

MILLET AND SORGHUM

FOREST

SPARSE VEGETATION

BANGLADESH

FOUR MAJOR FOOD GRAINS—rice, wheat, sorghum and millet—are grown for the most part in distinct regions of India according to climate, soil and custom. About 40 percent of the country's total land area is utilized for agriculture, which provides nearly half of the country's gross national product. In contrast, only about 20 percent of the land in the contiguous 48 states of the U.S. is devoted to growing crops. Yet the U.S., with a third of India's population, has nearly a third more cropland than India. India does, however, have the potential of irrigating much of its farmland to obtain two crops a year or even three. As the map suggests, the amount of land devoted to growing millet and sorghum (together with minor grains) exceeds the land planted to rice, which exceeds the land planted to wheat.

who will and who will not participate in a country's economic growth. The choice of a policy therefore involves a host of considerations.

It was neither accident nor ignorance that gave India a plan in the late 1950's and early 1960's that provided scant participation of the poor, little emphasis on agriculture and much emphasis on the growth of heavy industry. In the 1950's the essential ingredients of the "green revolution" were just emerging from agricultural research, and they offered no assurance that a heavy investment in agriculture would pay off.

Even though India did not make a single-minded commitment to the agricultural sector in the 1950's and 1960's, it had a generally fair record of growth, with regional high and low points and a good deal of experimentation. Perhaps the most interesting experiment was the massive Community Development Program. Initiated in 1952 in 25,000 villages, and by 1961 covering 500,000 villages and 300 million people, that program, with all its limitations, was among the first anywhere to take those integrated approaches that are currently fashionable among rural developers. The green revolution achieved its greatest success in the Punjab of northwestern India, which showed faster agricultural growth rates than Taiwan, often regarded as the model of agricultural success. (Taiwan and the Punjab have populations of nearly the same size.) Two other regions of India, parts of Gujarat in the west and Andhra in the south, also achieved striking agricultural production records in spite of having quite different cultural and institutional traditions. But India also includes Bihar, which has land-tenure customs that discourage increases in production, West Bengal, which combines great agricultural potential with low performance, and Madhya Pradesh, which has large areas with poor agricultural prospects. It is clearly difficult to generalize about the agriculture of a country whose regions exhibit such diversity. At the same time that diversity affords striking opportunities to make comparisons and draw lessons.

The growth of India's food-grain production in the two and a half decades since 1950 can be divided into three periods: a decade of accelerated growth based on traditional technology (1950–1960), a five-year period of transition (1960–1965) and a period of increasing dependence on new technology for raising production. The factors that accounted for the radical acceleration in grain production from the .11 percent rate of the colonial period to the 2.8 percent rate of the 1950's are hard to identify with precision. The burst of growth was clearly not due to investment in

modernization. To be sure, the use of fertilizer grew at a high rate, but it did so from an initial base that was close to zero. New crop varieties probably did little more than maintain yields in the face of diseases such as wheat rust. Moreover, there is scant evidence that the newly organized Community Development Program had an immediate impact on agricultural production.

Perhaps as much as a fifth of the production increase was due to the expansion of irrigation, some two-fifths to the increased utilization of labor associated with population growth and perhaps a third simply to increasing the amount of land under cultivation. The latter two factors and even the first can be attributed in large measure to new energies released and new incentives provided by national independence. An important stimulus was the reforms that removed the British system of collecting land taxes through a privileged group, whose members had become virtual lords of large estates.

India's creditable record of foodgrain production in the 1950's deteriorated in the early 1960's (on a weatheradjusted basis) to about 2 percent per year at the same time that population growth accelerated to nearly 2.5 percent per year and per capita incomes were rising at a higher rate than ever before. The rise in incomes was spurred by an industrial growth rate of almost 10 percent per year. Thus in spite of the fact that this was a brief period of increasing food aid from the U.S., food-grain prices rose faster than prices of other commodities. Partly as a result there was a slowing of industrial growth. This, combined with the disastrous drought of 1965–1967 and a precipitous decline in foreign aid, set the stage for a decade of overall economic stagnation.

Even as the pace of grain production was slackening, however, the prime movers of growth in agricultural output were shifting away from the forces associated with the end of colonial domination toward those associated with new technology. The bringing of new land under cultivation became less significant and the use of fertilizer became more so: the latter accounted for nearly 40 percent of the increase in grain production in the period 1961–1965, compared with less than 10 percent of the increase in the previous decade. Later the adoption of new high-yielding varieties of grain and new crop practices would increase the capacity of India's farms to absorb still more fertilizer, giving promise of further growth in the years ahead. Although the term green revolution was not yet current in 1961–1965, the institutional groundwork for the revolution was laid in those years.

Before the green revolution had ar-

rived, however, and almost as if to dramatize its urgency, the drought of 1965 cut grain production by 19 percent, or 17 million tons, canceling a full decade of grain-production growth. When the drought continued into the next year, with grain reserves wiped out, the hardship was immense, in spite of U.S. shipments of grain equal to almost 15 percent of India's diminished domestic production. Only the country's impressive capacity for operating relief programs averted a major disaster.

The influence of India's weather not only on Indian agriculture but also on how outside observers perceive the world food situation can hardly be exaggerated. In the years of good harvest in India (1949–1950, 1954–1955, 1961–1962, 1964–1965, 1970–1971 and 1975–1976) the world food situation has seemed bright and the talk has been of surpluses. In the years of poor harvest (1957–1958, 1965–1967 and 1972–1973) the situation has looked grim and the prophets of doom have been ascendant.

The first harvest after the drought, the harvest of 1968, showed a record-breaking gain in grain production of 28 percent in one year. The green revolution had arrived. Wheat production alone increased by five million tons and was to double over the next seven years, an average compound rate of growth of more than 10 percent per year. By the mid-1970's well over half of the land planted to "miracle" wheat varieties in the less developed countries was within the borders of India.

In India, however, the tonnage of wheat was then less than a third that of rice, and the impact of new technology was much less dramatic for rice than it was for wheat. The highly heterogeneous conditions of rice production make it much more difficult to breed successful new varieties. Moreover, the rice-growing regions of India have a less developed structure of supporting institutions than the wheat-growing ones. As a result the rice regions have lagged several years behind the wheat regions in benefiting from new technology.

Nevertheless, total grain production climbed at an average rate of 3.3 percent per year between the closely comparable and excellent weather years of 1964–1965 and 1970–1971. Sixty percent of the increase was attributable to the complex of factors associated with the intensified use of fertilizer. Because of the nature and the location of the new production the amount of grain reaching urban markets in the period from 1964–1965 to 1970–1971 accelerated at the impressive annual rate of 4.5 percent. In the short run this additional grain was used largely to displace imports, a strategy encouraged by the uncertain availability of U.S. supplies. In the long run the accelerated growth had profound implications for both the pace and the pattern of India's economic growth.

From 1971 to 1975 the growth of Indian grain production appeared to be stagnant. A series of droughts in 1972 and 1973 was quickly followed by a worldwide shortage of fertilizer caused by a worldwide lack of adequate fertilizer-production capacity and what can only be described as gross mismanagement of the worldwide fertilizer economy, particularly given the basic role of fertilizer in any effort to improve permanently the worldwide balance of food and population. This latter phenomenon hit hard exactly that aspect of the modernization of agriculture in which India's food hopes were necessarily being placed. The crop year 1975–

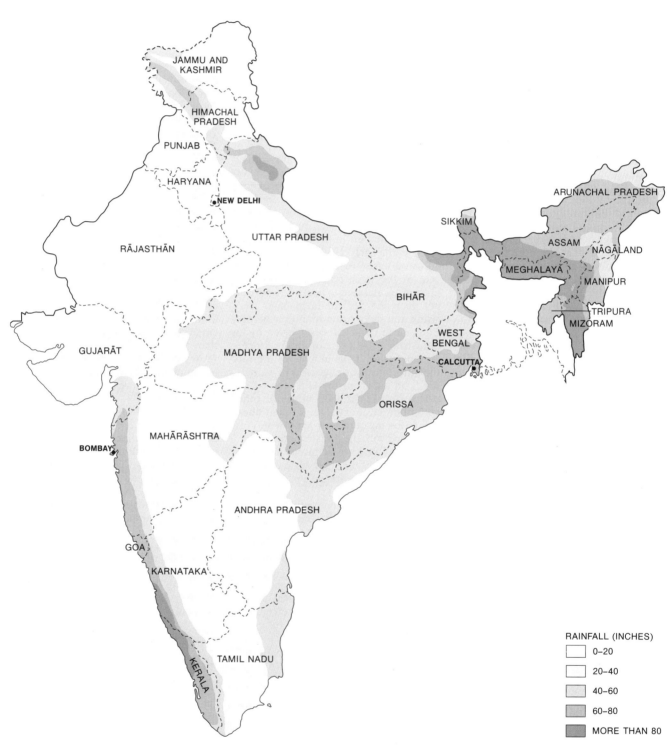

RAINFALL (INCHES)
- 0–20
- 20–40
- 40–60
- 60–80
- MORE THAN 80

PATTERN OF RAINFALL in India, as elsewhere, is a major determinant of crop selection and agricultural practices. The regions that receive from 40 to more than 80 inches of rainfall per year are favorable for growing rice (*see map on page 102*). Throughout most of India, from 75 to 90 percent of the the annual rainfall is concentrated during the four months of June, July, August and September, when India's weather is dominated by the rain-bearing winds of the southwest monsoon. Only the extreme northern and southern parts of the country receive a fairly uniform distribution of annual rainfall. A central problem of Indian agriculture is management of the water resources, including large and well-situated aquifers, for the years when the monsoon fails too provide the water for multiple cropping.

1976, however, with its good weather and the beginning of recovery in the availability of fertilizer, saw production jump to 116 million tons and food reserves increase by some 10 million tons. Whether or not India maintains and accelerates these agricultural growth rates depends on many complex factors and on the vigor with which new measures are pushed by the government and are accepted by the farmer.

One of the greatest problems that face the farmer, the agricultural statistician and the development planner is deciding whether or not a given change in technology or strategy is paying off. A change of a single percentage point in the growth rate of grain production can make an immense difference in the level of the minimum diet for millions of people and in determining the success of a development strategy. But how can one statistically detect a 1 percent change in the underlying trend when production has changed, as it has in India, by more than 10 percent in each year of six years of the past 25 and by more than 5 percent in more than half of the 25 years? Under such erratic conditions a judgment of a change in a trend cannot be based on standard statistical methods. About the best one can do is to try to match years of comparable weather and to trust that any difference in production can be attributed to policy and human effort.

The uncertainty faced by the statistician is of course an even more serious problem for the individual farmer. Judging whether an innovation will pay off is difficult enough after the fact. To judge the payoff before the fact is virtually impossible. Not only may the penalty for error be large but also it may be compounded by the random effects of the weather. The risk is further heightened if the farmer has little experience with recommendations from agricultural experiment stations and if the farm agent transmitting the advice is new at the job.

For the planner the year-to-year fluctuations in farm production are equally troubling as he tries to decide what level of foreign exchange to allocate for imports or what provisions, if any, to make for famine relief. Does he dare to increase employment, and hence the demand for food, by pushing an agriculture-based strategy, knowing that it may be politically irreversible? The reduction of the uncertainties that are the bane of agriculture calls for an enormous investment. The size of the investment may, in view of the magnitude of the uncertainties related to weather alone, dissuade the planner from following a strategy based on agriculture in favor of another kind of strategy that is stable but provides a slower growth in

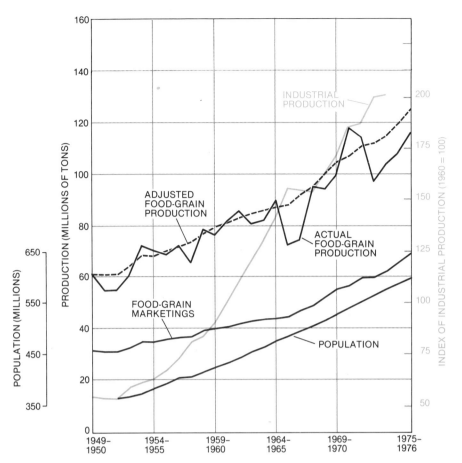

FOOD-GRAIN PRODUCTION IN INDIA has climbed, on the average, slightly faster than the population ever since India achieved independence in 1947. Because Indian agriculture depends heavily on the monsoon rains, however, there have been setbacks in years of deficient rainfall, notably 1965–1967 and 1972–1973. The curve labeled "Adjusted food-grain production" is a computed one that shows the production that could be expected from the known inputs of labor, fertilizer, seed varieties and so on, if weather conditions had been in the normal range. "Food-grain marketings" is also a computed curve, representing the grain available for sale in urban centers after allowance has been made for the grain consumed by the farm population. India's industrial growth since independence has been even more impressive than its agricultural performance, as is shown by the index of industrial production. In the future, however, India will at least have to modify its strategy of industrial growth if it is to finance the irrigation works and other costly facilities needed for its agriculture to develop adequately.

employment and incomes for the poor and a correspondingly slow growth in the demand for food.

Many people in developed countries still do not understand that the demand for food in developing countries is not rigidly linked to the laws of human biology. For countries such as India the demand is in large part the product of policies determining the choice of development strategy and the rate of employment growth and hence the fraction of the total income that is in the hands of the poor. Out of additions to income the laborers who constitute the bottom 20 percent on the income scale in India spend 60 percent on grain and 85 percent on agricultural commodities in general. The people in the top 10 percent on the income scale spend only 2 percent of additions to income on grain. Thus the effective demand for food depends significantly on who is receiving more

income. A high-employment strategy must be backed by a successful agricultural strategy.

The Indian election of 1971 is instructive on this point. In that year Mrs. Gandhi won a massive victory on the slogan of *garibi hatao*—abolish poverty. It was a slogan at least potentially appropriate to that year, when good weather and the green revolution combined for an extraordinarily large harvest. It proved not to be appropriate to the reality of the next five years, when the weather and external factors combined to stagnate agriculture and when the sharp decline in foreign assistance was retarding the growth of other sectors of the economy as well.

Thus there is a dilemma. On the one hand a strategy of growth oriented toward the reduction of poverty must, at least for a country of India's proportions, be based on accelerated growth in the agricultural sector. And that growth must be secured by countering fluctuations in the weather by a massive investment in assured irrigation and by certain access to foreign supplies of grain or the domestic storage of grain (with the consequent delay in the alleviation of poverty as the grain stocks are being built up). A strategy of poverty alleviation itself implies a political commitment and a restructuring of the political power base that cannot be reversed with a change in the weather.

On the other hand, a commitment to agriculture requires the allocation of resources on such a large scale as to preclude alternative strategies. India elected not to make a total commitment to agriculture in the late 1950's and early 1960's. Whether an agricultural strategy is chosen now depends on how the potential for success in agriculture is perceived; on the extent to which the world community chooses to assist in the realization of the agricultural potential and to provide guarantees against the vagaries of the weather; on whether the Indian world view sees national integrity

and dignity as lying with alleviating poverty or with strengthening the sinews of heavy industry, and on the realities of whether political power will be maintained on the basis of appeal to a coalition of the highly organized upper-income civil-service class and the wealthy big-business interests or appeal to the less organized but more numerous poor. Hence the rate of growth in food production is an interactive result of a basic political decision and a choice of an overall strategy of development. Only after these decisions are made do the details of agricultural production strategy become relevant and operational.

The potential role of foreign assistance and other external factors in the choice of a development strategy is also illuminated by the events of this period. In 1965 foreign assistance represented more than 20 percent of India's gross investment. By 1972 that aid had dropped to zero in terms of actual net resource transfers, with a consequent sharp drop in real investment and in government revenues. After 1972 the

total of foreign assistance increased again, but it increased by less than the huge, price-induced rise in the bill for imported food and oil. Thus just when crops were poor, the resources to finance the importation of food and the goods needed for development were sharply reduced. Compounding the problem, the grain stocks built in the first flush of the green revolution were wiped out by the temporary but heavy impact of some 10 million refugees from Bangladesh, of the enormous rise in grain prices following the dramatic move of the U.S.S.R. into world grain markets in 1973 and of the drought in 1974. It is no wonder that Mrs. Gandhi could not deliver on her promises and has had to reexamine the basis of her 1971 political strategy.

Not only are agriculture and income linked but also both are closely bound to population growth. It is still thought by many, particularly in developed countries, that the obvious way for a country such as India to win the food-population race is simply to reduce the fertility rate of its people. It is now clear, however, that the extent to which birthrates decline is a function of how broadly the population participates in economic and social benefits. And, for the reasons I have outlined, that participation is a function of the extent to which agricultural growth can be accelerated to meet the food demands associated with a growth in employment.

It is now well documented that in economic systems providing broad participation, such as those in Taiwan, China, Sri Lanka (formerly Ceylon) and the state of Kerala in India birthrates may decline sooner and at lower levels of average income than one would have predicted from the experience of Western Europe and the U.S. Although family-planning efforts deserve credit for an important assist, there is little evidence to support the view that such efforts, even with subtle (and not so subtle) forms of persuasion, can succeed alone. Hence the paradox: more food production now is necessary for the decline in fertility that will reduce the pressures to increase food production later.

After more than two decades of gradual evolution in India and elsewhere the broad outlines of a successful rural strategy are clearly evident. What is less clear are the details of implementation and the probable quantitative successes of the strategy.

One can say with some confidence that India has the potential to accelerate its agricultural growth to a rate of 3.5 to 4 percent per year. Indeed, such estimates actually leave a margin for error and underfulfillment. To enumerate the requisites for such growth is to illumi-

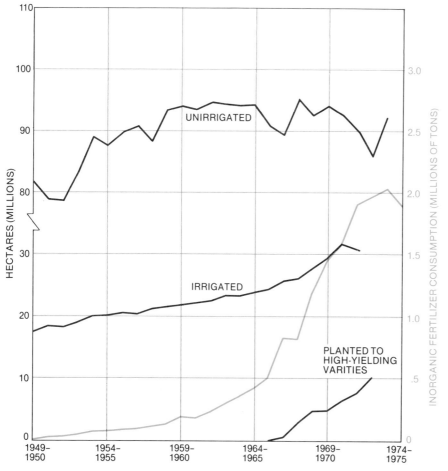

ESSENTIALS OF THE "GREEN REVOLUTION" in India are inorganic fertilizers, irrigation and new high-yielding varieties of grains. Indian agriculture has always depended heavily on irrigation. Even in 1950 nearly one hectare in five planted to food grains was irrigated; today one hectare in four is under irrigation. In the U.S. less than 5 percent of all farmland requires irrigation. Between 1959 and 1974 use of inorganic fertilizer in India rose at a rate of 19 percent per year. India uses a seventh as much fertilizer per hectare of farmland as U.S.

nate the risks and the underlying dilemma. The requisites fall into four categories: massive investment in irrigation, power and transportation; huge increases in fertilizer supplies; effective organization of agricultural research, and widespread improvement of institutions for rural development (including the difficult-to-orchestrate participation of the small farmer). Regionally the key to short-term success rests heavily in the states that lie on the fertile plain in the eastern downstream reaches of the Ganges. These, however, are the states with institutional foundations that are less well developed for agricultural growth than the average for the country. Politically the key to success is a decentralization of decision making, with all the risks attendant on building new bases of political power. The necessary reallocation of resources will weaken the political bond to traditional groups while creating the potential for support from new groups. It is no wonder that the simplistic advice of outside observers for raising production (for example "Get your prices right") is viewed with disdain by those wrestling with the actuality of achieving growth in agriculture in India.

The accelerated growth of Indian agriculture depends fundamentally on the development of new varieties of high-yielding crops. These in turn will provide their maximum benefits only with assured supplies of water and fertilizer. The transportation of fertilizer and other farm inputs, and the resulting increased output, calls for further investment in vehicles and roads.

The rapid increase in grain production in the late 1960's was achieved in large part through the expansion of irrigation, which required a big investment not only in conventional irrigation works but also in electric power to operate the pumps needed for well irrigation in the responsive wheat areas of the northwest. Comparable agricultural growth can be extended eastward on the Gangetic Plain with high-yielding varieties of rice, assuming that abundant groundwater resources are tapped to supplement the monsoon rains. If water is made available, an irrigated wheat crop can be planted after each rice harvest. That development is already in progress, proving its potential, but it has a long way to go. The added investment required will be even larger than the one made in the late 1960's. Even in that period large tonnages of potential wheat output were lost because of power shortages, particularly in dry years, when deficits of water curtailed the electric power for irrigation pumps.

The fertilizer requirements for the accelerated growth of farm output are also immense: annual growth rates of 15 to 20 percent, annual increments

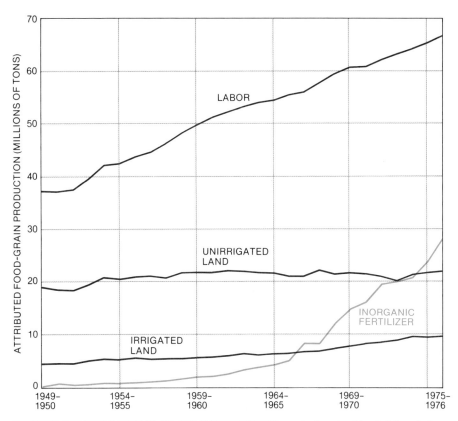

FACTORS DETERMINING GRAIN PRODUCTION are the inputs of land, labor, irrigation and fertilizer. The curves show how the rising Indian production of food grains can be allocated among the four inputs. Over the entire 29-year period since independence the biggest factor in raising grain output has been the increasing input of labor, an increase made possible by, as well as necessitated by, the increase in the population of the country. In the past decade, however, the increased use of inorganic fertilizer has added as much to grain output as was added by increased inputs of labor over the past two decades. The effect of high-yielding varieties of grain is manifested principally in the curve given for fertilizer. Sum of four curves corresponds to the curve labeled "Adjusted food-grain production" in illustration on page 105.

of 200,000 to 400,000 tons of nitrogen alone, representing hundreds of millions of dollars of investment per year, compounded at staggering rates. Such a prodigious investment for fertilizer may clash with the rest of the agricultural-growth strategy, let alone with a capital-intensive industrial-growth one. The alternative of importing fertilizer raises all the hard political questions presented by dependency on outside sources of supply. It is out of such enormously complex considerations that development dilemmas are made. Achieving high rates of growth in agriculture is not just a matter of knowing what to do to raise farm output; it quickly involves problems of national independence, guesses about the volume of aid that may be expected from other countries and sharp shifts in political constituencies and loyalties, depending on the growth strategy chosen.

If agricultural success in India, and elsewhere, depends fundamentally on new crop varieties, it is clear that they must be developed within the country for which they are intended. They can rarely be transferred from the very different conditions of California, Iowa, Mexico or the Philippines. India's peasants have evolved highly effective production and storage methods, well suited to India's wide diversity of environments. Successful change is not to be sought in changing the peasants' wise and perceptive minds but rather in changing the environment within which the peasants make their decisions. To effect such a change a complex institutional structure combining research and local services must be built. Great strides in filling this need were made in the late 1950's with assistance from the Rockefeller Foundation, which drew on experience gained from effective work in Mexico and elsewhere. The institutional structure needs further strengthening and continued interaction with such centers of excellence as the International Rice Research Institute in the Philippines. Unfortunately the structure is still weakest in the part of the rice area that has the greatest immediate physical potential.

The implementation of policies to spread new agricultural technologies requires a comprehensive system of institutions for distributing fertilizer, teach-

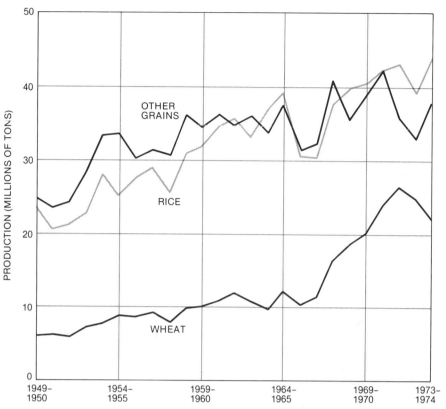

PRODUCTION OF RICE AND WHEAT in India has been increasing more rapidly than the production of other food grains. The sharp rise in wheat production reflects the adoption of high-yielding varieties. The introduction of new rice varieties has proceeded more slowly, in part because more rice varieties are needed to suit India's highly heterogeneous conditions.

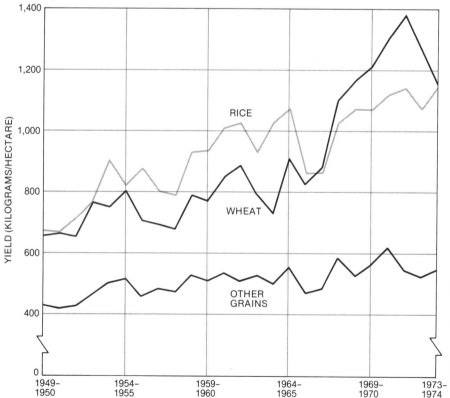

COMPARISON OF YIELDS shows rice and wheat far ahead of other food grains. Over the 24-year period plotted the yield of rice has shown a fairly steady increase of about 3 percent per year. There was not much improvement in the yield of wheat until the new high-yielding varieties appeared in the late 1960's. The sharp drop in wheat yields after 1972 was due to a shortage of fertilizer combined with a shortage of water for irrigation. The shortage of irrigation water was largely attributable to a lack of energy for pumps. The yield of other food grains is considerably lower than it is for wheat and rice and will be difficult to improve in the future.

ing new methods, providing credit, organizing knowledge of individual regions and marketing farm output. Such institutions must be staffed by trained personnel and are unlikely to work effectively unless farmers are literate enough not only to grasp and exploit what the institutions have to offer so that they perform effectively and efficiently but also to influence the institutions and the formally educated people who run them. Hence a broadly based educational system is also an important ingredient of agricultural growth. Although the number of boys aged six to 10 enrolled in the primary schools of India increased from 60 to 99 percent between 1951 and 1965, and the proportion of girls enrolled increased from 25 to 56 percent, the overall educational base remains narrow and continues to act as a brake on growth in farm output.

The task of effecting change is complicated by the fact that the farms accounting for a fourth of the agricultural land in India are smaller than two hectares (five acres). The very small farmers are poor and are wary of experimentation. If they can be persuaded to innovate and if they are serviced with the necessary institutions, however, they are at least as effective in their use of fertilizers, pesticides and water as farmers with larger holdings. Carrying the message of new technologies to the small farmer and integrating them into the credit, marketing and educational institutions also require a costly investment in trained personnel.

India has gone far in two decades, in building farm-centered institutions, in experimenting with community development, in creating the Intensive Agricultural District Program and the Small Farmers' Development Agency, in establishing cooperative credit unions and rural banks and more. The substantial success of such ventures provides a firm base for optimism. There is nonetheless still much to be done, and it requires time and the careful assignment of priorities at a high level in the society. The success of the past effort must be seen in the perspective of an initially very low base of accomplishment at the time of independence, and the scale of that effort is indicative of the additional effort needed if the large remaining potentials of Indian agriculture are to be realized.

The region with probably the greatest potential for agricultural growth lies on the eastern Gangetic Plain, where four principal states produced 22 percent of India's grain in 1970–1971 while accounting for only 10 percent of the country's consumption of nitrogenous fertilizer. The region is richly endowed with groundwater. The principal brake on its agricultural growth has been its failure to develop adequate institutions of the type I have been describing.

In West Bengal, a key state in the region, much of the land is held by a system of petty landlords that probably inhibits the institutional development crucial to agricultural modernization. The landlords typically each own an average of about four hectares, worked by three or four tenants and their families. There are of course a great many landlords. In neither a Western-style democracy nor a more centralized regime is a landlord class of this size to be treated lightly in the political process. Can it be reformed now by legislation securing tenancy and fixing rents? Is a more radical land reform possible? Can production be increased without reform? If production increases, will underlying social tensions become so exacerbated as to upset the political stability necessary for continued gains? The questions are familiar to those in power. The answers come easily—to those without responsibility for the consequences. From such complexity arises indecision that is all the greater when the resources are so limited and the political risks so great.

Beyond the political problem lies the uncertainty about how best to build institutions: by extension of the better institutions from other states or by the slower and more acceptable process of reforming existing structures within the state. If it is the latter, one must work with the full knowledge that the present structures are deficient precisely because of the flaws in existing political and institutional relations.

In the face of such complexity and uncertainty, what may one expect for a growth rate in Indian agriculture? If irrigation expands at the high rate of the period 1961–1968, if the use of fertilizer expands at nearly as high a rate as it did in the same period, if agricultural researchers come up with the improved varieties and practices, particularly for rice, that are essential to the profitable application of irrigation and fertilizer, if the efforts to reach the small farmer succeed, then a growth rate approaching 5 percent is plausible. If the 3.3 percent growth rate of 1965 to 1971 qualified as a green revolution, 5 percent is a grand prospect indeed. If one makes a somewhat more conservative estimate of the response to the physical inputs, say the actual response of the 1950's, the agricultural growth rate should still reach 4 percent. The underlying quantities projected for each of the inputs are reasonable; that they should all be achieved simultaneously is perhaps not. With allowances for shortfalls a growth rate of 3.5 to 4 percent seems a safe projection. Such a growth rate in agriculture is consistent with an overall strategy that would provide accelerated growth in industry and a broadly participatory pattern of development. An increase in food-grain production of half a percentage point may seem small, but it is not when it is applied to such a large and basic sector or when it is seen in terms of

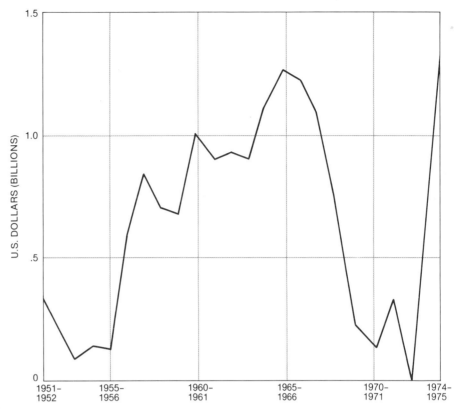

FOREIGN AID FOR INDIA increased rather steadily from the mid-1950's to the mid-1960's, then plunged sharply. The figures plotted here represent net foreign-resource transfers to India's account, computed as the difference between what India had to pay for imports and what the country earned from exports. The sharp rise in these net foreign-resource transfers in the past few years reflects the steep increase in the cost of imported oil and fertilizer.

the actual improvement in diet and reduction in human misery.

One can see that the extent to which India accelerates agricultural production is in large part a political choice involving both internal and external considerations. Four aspects subject to foreign influence are of importance. First, assistance in the form of grain or credits can ensure basic supplies of food in the face of fluctuating weather conditions and lags in production. Such a food-security system, backed by the international community, may encourage the shift to a rural, employment-oriented strategy.

Second, foreign technical assistance in research, education and many other aspects of rural development can lessen the constraint on growth that would otherwise be set by the shortage of trained personnel. The level of assistance must be skillfully measured because the objective is to accelerate the immediate performance of the needed tasks without delaying India's long-term capacity to perform the tasks by itself. Since India now has the basic agricultural institutions in place and a large corps of highly skilled and experienced administrators, it is quite able to effectively absorb assistance in clearly defined technical areas.

Third, financial assistance on a major scale can not only relieve the capital requirements of rural growth but also meet the crucial need for foreign exchange while the Indian economy adjusts to the more favorable environment for the export of labor-intensive modern industrial and processed goods, which is implicit in the new strategy.

Fourth, and perhaps most important, is an international environment that gives first priority to the humane aspects of development rather than to gaining short-term political advantages in the arena of great-power politics. Although in the long run the rural-oriented strategy has a greater potential for faster growth than the alternative urban-industrial strategy, in the short run it calls for a greater dependence on others for food, fertilizer, technology and capital. Certainly the sharp decline in net foreign aid to India from $1.2 billion in 1965 ($2.63 per capita) to essentially nil in 1972 argues against increased dependence on Western countries and hence for a more cautious, narrowly based and inward-looking approach to growth. Political success tends to be judged on the short run, and politicians frequently choose strategies of growth that maximize short-term security at the expense of long-term security. Before other countries judge India's decisions they should examine their own short- and long-term priorities. It is not only the world view of India's leaders that is being tested.

10

The Resources Available
for Agriculture

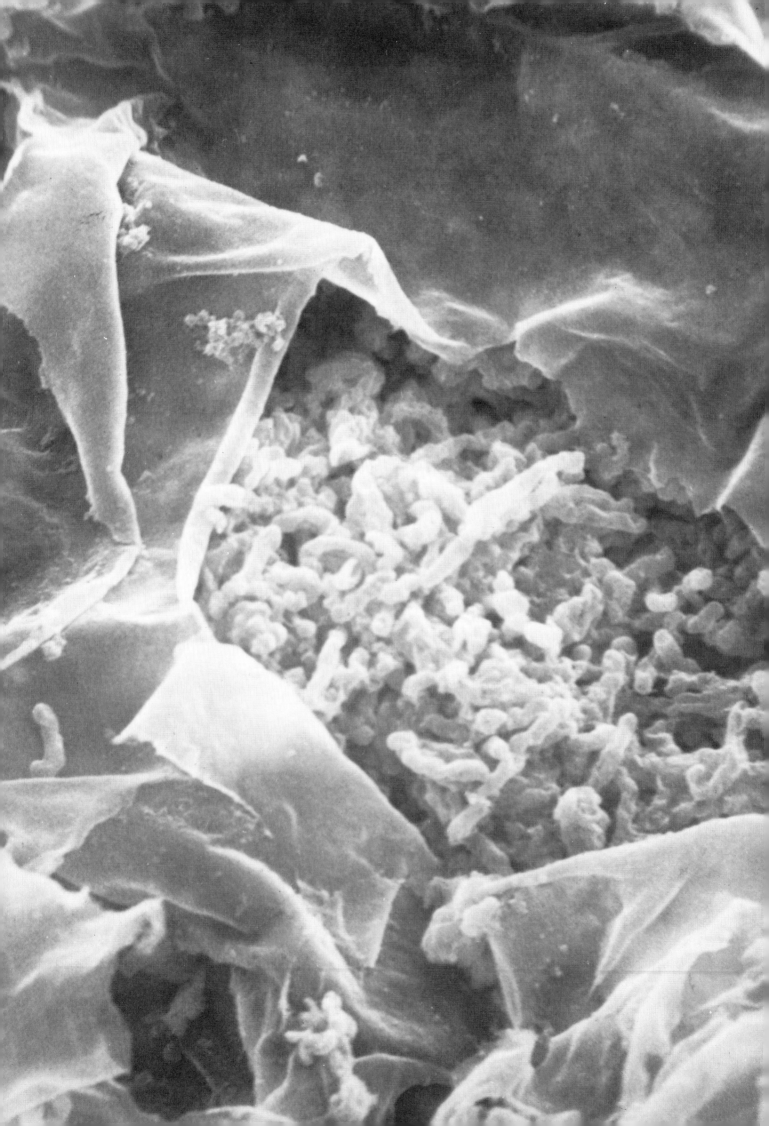

The Resources Available for Agriculture

ROGER REVELLE

The physical resources of earth, air, fire (energy) and water are large but are essentially fixed. The biological and social resources, however, are far from being pressed to the limit.

In considering the resources required to supply food for human beings we tend to think of the resources used directly in agriculture. Only a portion of the food products grown by farmers, however, can be eaten without further processing. Most farm products must be stored, transported, distributed and cooked before they can contribute to human nutrition. Thus we need to think of the resources necessary for the entire human food system and not only of the resources utilized by farmers.

We should remember also the other ways, actual or potential, in which human beings can obtain food supplies. Long ago, before the invention of agriculture, men and women worked for their living very much as other animals do, by gathering the edible portions of wild plants and invertebrate animals, by hunting and by fishing. The resources required were few and simple: flints and other workable stones for spear points and arrowheads, plant fibers for fishnets and containers, clay for ceramic pots, wood for cooking and bones for tools and fishhooks.

The world's fisheries are the modern counterpart of this ancient method of food production. They provide about 10 percent of the protein available to the present world population (and a much higher percentage in many poor countries) but only a small part of total food energy. These proportions are likely to diminish in the future. The maximum sustainable fish catch is probably not more than twice the present one, and the resources required for attaining this maximum, particularly the requirements for fuel energy, are high. The situation might be changed by the development of "mariculture," or ocean farming, but this approach is not likely to add substantially to the food supply in the foreseeable future.

If the world's human population of between six and seven billion in the year 2000—let alone the larger population that can be expected 50 to 100 years from today—is to be adequately fed, a massive increase in agricultural production will be necessary. Whether and how this can be brought about depends on the magnitude of the resources available to farmers and on the efficiency with which they are able to use them. The resources fall into two broad categories: natural (including physical and biological resources) and social.

The physical resources, although they are very large, are ultimately fixed; they are the four basic elements of the Greeks: earth, air, fire and water. (Our modern metaphor for *pyr*, the fire of the Greeks, is the Greek word for work: *energeia*, or energy.) The biological resources, on the other hand, cannot be assigned dimensions or limits; they include the plants and animals farmers grow and the microbes and other organisms that play diverse roles in the food system. The social resources are also basically unbounded; they include the capital for agricultural investment, the social institutions that help the farmers to do their job, human labor and skills, and the growing store of scientific and practical knowledge that has transformed agriculture in the past and can be counted on to cause even greater changes in the future.

Thomas Malthus' "principle of population" states that human populations will always increase up to a limit set by human food supplies. Malthus thought this limit was determined by the physical resources available for agriculture. He recognized that farm production increases with improved technology, and that the stock of usable resources can also be made to increase. He believed, however, that the rates of increase would always be less than the potential capacity of human beings to multiply their numbers. These ideas about the relation between population and resources still underlie much contemporary thought. Here I shall look at the inverse of Malthus' proposition: Can the effective utilization of resources for food production be made to increase to limits set by human population size? A more important question is: Can rates of growth of agricultural production be made to exceed rates of population growth, thereby improving the conditions of life of poor people throughout the world? Such improvement is probably one of the essential conditions for reducing birthrates and eventually stopping population growth.

The physical resources of the food system need to be defined more narrowly than simply as being those things in the environment that can be utilized with currently available technology. The concept of a resource carries with it the qualities of scarcity and value. Choices must be made about the uses to which a resource will be put, because it does not exist in sufficient quantity to be used for all possible purposes. In this sense only some of the factors of physical production in agriculture can be

NITROGEN-FIXING MICROORGANISMS supply about two-thirds of the fixed nitrogen used worldwide by growing crops. One of most important nitrogen-fixing bacteria is *Rhizobium japonicum*, which converts atmospheric nitrogen into ammonia in the root nodules of soybeans. The soybean incorporates the ammonia into nucleic acids, proteins and chlorophyll. The scanning electron micrograph on the opposite page shows *Rhizobium* bacteria released when a soybean nodule cell was slit open. Bacteria are the puffy structures. The micrograph, enlarged about 2,900 diameters, was made by Winston J. Brill of the University of Wisconsin.

thought of as resources. For example, sunlight and carbon dioxide are fundamental for photosynthesis but they are not scarce, and the quantities available cannot be changed very much or allocated by deliberate human action. Only about one part in 200,000 of the sunlight falling on the earth is converted into food energy for human beings, and only about three parts in 10,000 of the atmospheric carbon dioxide are temporarily utilized each year in human metabolism and returned again to the air.

Human beings are inadvertently increasing the carbon dioxide content of the atmosphere by burning coal, oil and natural gas, and in the process they may be reducing the incoming sunlight, by increasing the area covered by clouds. If present trends in the use of fossil fuels continue, the carbon dioxide content of

the air may increase five- or sixfold in the next 100 years. The effects on the world's climate are quite uncertain, but they may cause serious disruptions in the food system. It is certain, however, that the efficiency of photosynthesis, that is, the portion of the incoming solar radiation that plants can convert into chemical energy, will be considerably increased, perhaps almost in direct proportion to the rise in atmospheric carbon dioxide, if, as some experiments indicate, the limiting factor in photosynthetic production under otherwise good environmental conditions is the availability of carbon dioxide.

Molecular nitrogen and oxygen, the two major constituents of the air, are essential for plant metabolism but in their atmospheric form they, like carbon dioxide, cannot be thought of as re-

sources because they have no economic value. The respiration of all the plants and animals on the earth utilizes only about one part in 5,000 of the earth's oxygen each year and nearly all of it is returned promptly to the air in the process of photosynthesis. All biological processes together probably utilize less than a millionth of the atmospheric nitrogen, and it too is returned to the air through complex bacterial action. The biological and chemical processes by which the molecular nitrogen in the atmosphere is "fixed," that is, combined with other elements into substances that can be metabolized by plants, do, however, utilize resources in the sense we have defined.

The other physical resources—earth, water and energy—are relatively limited in quantity and have economic value;

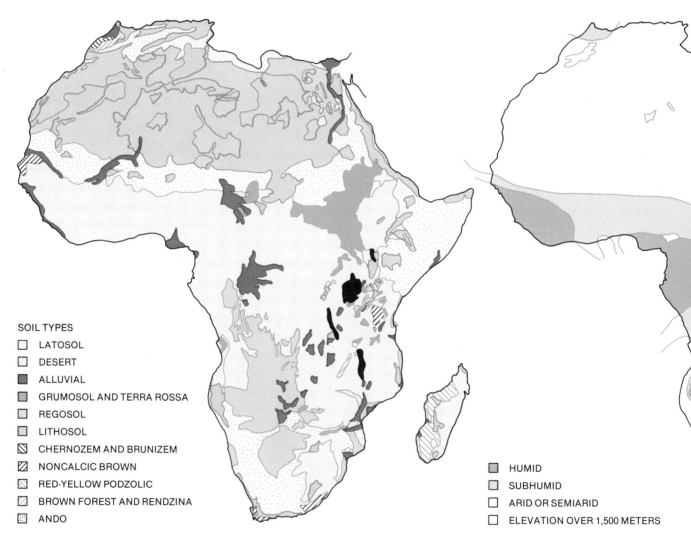

SOIL TYPES
☐ LATOSOL
⬚ DESERT
⬛ ALLUVIAL
▨ GRUMOSOL AND TERRA ROSSA
▥ REGOSOL
▦ LITHOSOL
▨ CHERNOZEM AND BRUNIZEM
▨ NONCALCIC BROWN
▧ RED-YELLOW PODZOLIC
▨ BROWN FOREST AND RENDZINA
▦ ANDO

▨ HUMID
☐ SUBHUMID
☐ ARID OR SEMIARID
☐ ELEVATION OVER 1,500 METERS

SOIL AND CLIMATE OF AFRICA point up some of the limitations placed on agricultural development even in parts of the world where temperature, sunlight and, in some regions, precipitation are otherwise favorable. Africa, including Madagascar, contains about 23 percent of the world's land area not covered by ice. Although Africa is representative of the world at large in that about a fifth of its land area is considered potentially arable, or cultivable, its principal soil types are among the least favorable for agriculture (map at left). Five soil groups, the first five listed in the key, make up 96 percent of the potentially arable land. One-third of Africa is covered by latosol, the reddish soil of tropical forests, of which less than half could be used for growing crops. Because latosols are the most highly leached soils in the world, they require chemical fertilizers and a variety of minerals to be agriculturally productive. Fifty-seven percent of the potentially arable soil in Africa is latosol. Next most abundant potentially arable soil, nearly 20 percent of the total, consists of desert soil, which is also deficient in many plant nutrients. Regosol, a sandy, undifferentiated soil, represents 6.4 percent of the total potentially

they must be allocated among different uses by deliberate human action. By the earth we mean in agricultural terms primarily arable land—land areas covered with soil in which crops can be grown—and grazing land on which livestock can feed. The earth also contains deposits of rocks high in phosphates, potash and metals, which can be mined and converted into plant nutrients and into farm tools and machinery.

Water is part of the chemical substrate for photosynthesis. It is utilized by food crops, however, principally for cooling and as a medium for the transport of substances between different parts of the growing plant. Since the transport is driven by differential vapor pressures, it results in a high rate of evapotranspiration from the leaves. For example, wheat, rice and corn commonly evapotranspire thousands of tons of water per ton of edible grain produced. Most of the water used deliberately by human beings is devoted to agriculture, and for many of the world's peoples water is a scarce resource.

The most important type of energy utilized in agriculture is sunlight, which is converted into chemical energy in the process of photosynthesis. Only a small fraction of the solar energy irradiating crop plants, usually less than 1 percent, is utilized in the manufacture of substances that can serve as food for human beings. Perhaps the most fundamental problem of agricultural research is to increase this fraction.

No plant or animal is able to fix nitrogen, only prokaryotes: organisms, including bacteria and blue-green algae, that have no cell nuclei. In legumes part of the solar energy captured by photosynthesis is transferred in the form of carbohydrates to symbiotic bacteria called rhizobia, which use it to make ammonia from atmospheric nitrogen and the hydrogen in carbohydrates. This fixed nitrogen is in turn utilized by the plants to make chlorophyll, nucleic acids and proteins. Other bacteria utilize the energy in organic waste to fix nitrogen. In the blue-green algae the photosynthetic conversion of solar energy and the fixation of atmospheric nitrogen occur in the same organism.

In modern high-yielding agriculture the biological fixation processes do not provide enough nitrogen for maximum production of nonleguminous crops. Hence chemical nitrogen fertilizers, in which the energy for nitrogen fixation is supplied by natural gas or other fossil

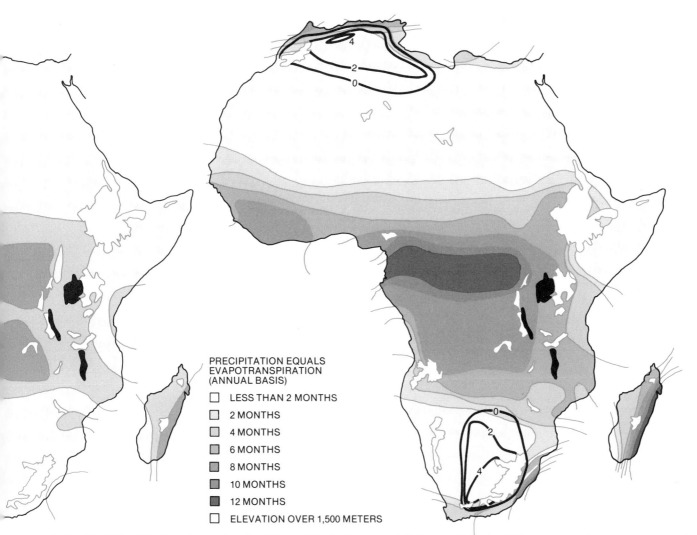

PRECIPITATION EQUALS
EVAPOTRANSPIRATION
(ANNUAL BASIS)

☐ LESS THAN 2 MONTHS
☐ 2 MONTHS
☐ 4 MONTHS
☐ 6 MONTHS
☐ 8 MONTHS
☐ 10 MONTHS
☐ 12 MONTHS
☐ ELEVATION OVER 1,500 METERS

arable land in Africa; it holds water poorly unless it is specially treated. Grumosol and terra rossa, which together make up about 7 percent of the arable total, present lesser problems. Only 7 percent of the arable land in Africa consists of naturally rich alluvial soil. The second great agricultural deficiency of Africa is poor distribution of rainfall. More than half of Africa is arid or semiarid (*map in middle*). To support agriculture such areas would have to import water from outside sources during all or part of the year. In subhumid regions the annual precipitation exceeds evaporation, but some runoff of precipitation must be stored if crops are to be grown year round. Only in the humid areas can crops be grown without irrigation in all months when the average minimum temperature is above freezing. The limitation that lack of water places on agricultural development is shown in the map at the right, depicting the number of months per year in which precipitation plus residual soil moisture would exceed the potential evapotranspiration of crops. Black contour lines indicate regions where frost is likely; associated numbers give number of months when average minimum temperature falls below freezing.

fuels, must be used. Both the natural bacterial process and the chemical manufacturing process apparently require about the same amount of energy per unit of fixed nitrogen produced: roughly 15,000 kilocalories per kilogram. In the symbiotic bacterial process the energy is supplied by the plant's own synthetic product, which may explain why the yields per hectare of soybeans and other seed legumes are comparatively low. For every ton of soybeans, containing 30 to 40 percent protein, 100 kilograms of nitrogen must be fixed by the symbiotic rhizobia, which in the process consume the energy in 400 kilograms of carbohydrate. Because of the high energy content of natural gas and naphtha, the fossil fuels commonly used in chemical nitrogen fixation, only about 150 kilograms of fuel is consumed to provide 100 kilograms of nitrogen in the form of chemical nitrogen fertilizer. Even at current oil and gas prices the cost of this quantity of fossil fuel is less than 10 percent of the value of the resulting crop yield.

In world agriculture as a whole synthetically fixed nitrogen represents only about 30 percent of the total fixed nitrogen metabolized by crop plants. Forty million tons of synthetically fixed nitrogen were applied worldwide in 1974. According to estimates by Ralph W. F. Hardy of E. I. du Pont de Nemours & Company, among others, the annual biological fixation in agricultural soil amounts to about 90 million tons: 35 million tons in crop legumes, nine million tons in nonlegume food crops and 45 million tons in permanent meadows and grasslands. Probably another 45 million tons of atmospheric nitrogen are fixed annually by lightning, by the action of ozone and by combustion, including forest fires, and part of this nitrogen is deposited on the earth's farmlands. It is estimated that by the year 2000, 160 million tons of chemically fixed nitrogen—four times as much as in 1974—will be used in world agriculture, requiring 250 to 300 million tons of fossil fuels. This corresponds to roughly 4 percent of present fuel consumption. At 1976 prices of $200 to $250 per ton of fixed nitrogen the cost of nitrogen fertilizer would be $32 billion to $40 billion, of which the fossil-fuel cost would be $15 billion to $20 billion. That would still be a small fraction of the estimated $300-billion value of the crop production that is attributable to the application of fertilizer.

Mechanical energy is needed in agriculture to lift water for irrigation, to cultivate, plant and harvest the fields, to transport farm inputs and products and for many other purposes. In traditional agriculture most of the mechanical energy is provided by the labor of human beings and animals; in modern agriculture the primary energy source is usually fossil fuels or hydroelectric power. David Pimentel and his colleagues at Cornell University have shown that where chemical fertilizers and farm machinery, including pumps for irrigation, are utilized efficiently in the modern agriculture of the developed countries, the total fossil-fuel energy required to produce food grains—the primary agricultural product in most of the world—is about half the energy in the seeds of the grain. In the developed countries, however, animal products, including meat, eggs, milk, butter and cheese, are major components of the food system. Animals convert only 10 to 20 percent of the energy in their feed into the energy contained in edible products; moreover, considerable energy must be expended in animal care and maintenance. Hence, as Pimentel has emphasized, the energy invested in producing milk, eggs and meat in the agriculture of the developed countries is often several times greater than the energy contained in the edible products.

The present high prices and foreseeable exhaustion of fossil fuels raise serious questions of whether the energy-intensive agriculture of the developed countries can be extended to other parts of the world or can even be continued for very long in any country. In principle, however, most—perhaps all—of the energy needed in modern high-yielding agriculture could be provided by the farmers themselves. For every ton of cereal grain there are one to two tons of humanly inedible crop residues with an energy content considerably greater than the food energy in the grain. If only half of this energy could be recovered by the fermentative production of methane or alcohol, the energy requirement for modern agriculture, including ener-

	NET ARABLE AREA IN HUMID TROPICS (MILLIONS OF HECTARES)	ARABLE WITHOUT IRRIGATION OUTSIDE HUMID TROPICS (MILLIONS OF HECTARES)	IRRIGATION REQUIRED FOR EVEN ONE CROP (MILLIONS OF HECTARES)	GROSS CROPPED AREA WITHOUT IRRIGATION (MILLIONS OF HECTARES)	GROSS CROPPED AREA ADDED BY IRRIGATION (MILLIONS OF HECTARES)	TOTAL POTENTIAL GROSS CROPPED AREA (MILLIONS OF HECTARES)
AFRICA	105	490	10	705	290	995
ASIA	80	450	15	625	475	1,100
AUSTRALIA, NEW ZEALAND	0	115	2	123	2	125
EUROPE	0	170	0	205	40	245
NORTH AMERICA	10	440	8	535	160	695
SOUTH AMERICA	300	350	24	635	80	715
U.S.S.R.	0	325	23	325	30	355
TOTAL	495	2,340	82	3,155	1,077	4,230

POTENTIALLY ARABLE LAND capable of supporting crops without irrigation constitutes some 22 percent of the world's ice-free land surface. About 495 million hectares lie within the humid Tropics, 2,340 million hectares lie outside. Water is available to irrigate another 80-odd million hectares, which then can produce one crop a year. Omitting arable land for which no water is available (about 200 million hectares worldwide), the ratio of potentially arable land to total land in Africa, Asia and North America is typical of the world as a whole: about one hectare in five. In Australia, New Zealand and the U.S.S.R. the proportion is less: about one hectare in six or seven. In Europe, however, more than one hectare in three is arable, and in South America the proportion approaches two in five. Where climatic conditions allow, more than one crop a year can be grown. Columns labeled "Gross cropped areas" indicate the potential; the figures represent potentially arable land multiplied by number of crops that could be grown in a four-month growing season.

gy for the production of chemical fertilizers, could be fully satisfied.

In both traditional and modern food systems the energy expended in food processing, distribution and cooking is much greater than the energy expended in food production. For example, in rural India about twice as much fuel energy is used in cooking a kilogram of rice as there is food energy in the rice. In the U.S., estimates by John S. Steinhart of the University of Wisconsin and Carol E. Steinhart, when combined with Pimentel's figure for farm energy expenditures, show that twice as much energy is consumed outside the farms in processing, packaging, transporting, distributing, refrigerating and cooking food as the farmers consume in growing it. In both countries the energy requirement for the entire food system could, in the long run, present more serious problems than meeting the energy needs for crop production.

The three biological factors of importance in agriculture are, first, the gene pools of crop plants and domestic animals; second, various kinds of microorganisms, and third, earthworms, insects and other larger organisms that turn over and aerate the soil. Only a tiny fraction of the living species of plants and animals have been domesticated to play a role in the human food system: primarily cereal and leguminous food grains, certain tubers and a relatively small number of vegetables, fruits and nuts among the plants; ruminants, swine and poultry among the animals. These few domesticated species have become highly specialized through many generations of controlled breeding. They are vastly different from their wild ancestors, particularly in their vulnerability to diseases and pests. One of the major problems of modern agriculture is to retain a sufficient diversity in the gene pools of domestic species and to preserve the genes of their wild relatives, in order to allow breeding of new varieties resistant to mutant disease organisms and resurgent pests as they appear in different parts of the world.

In addition to the nitrogen-fixing bacteria and blue-green algae other microorganisms of vital importance in the world food system are the bacterial flora in the rumen of cattle, sheep and goats; soil microbes, both fungi and bacteria, that perform a variety of functions, and microorganisms that can be employed to process foods by fermentation. One of the most remarkable symbiotic associations in human affairs is that between men, ruminant animals and the rumen bacteria. The bacteria are able to convert cellulose, which human beings cannot metabolize, into the sugars and carbohydrates that they can. The bacteria also manufacture amino acids, the subunits of proteins, from simple nitrogen compounds. As a result the ruminants can provide nutritious human food from a diet of grasses, leaves, organic wastes and even human and animal excreta, along with certain simple compounds, such as urea. In traditional agriculture and pastoralism ruminants also represent a means of storing and transporting food supplies. Moreover, they provide much of the mechanical energy for cultivating the fields.

One gram of fertile soil may contain tens of thousands of protozoan and algal cells, a million fungal cells and more than 10 million bacteria. It has long been known that enzymes and acids manufactured by the bacteria release phosphates and other plant nutrients from soil minerals, but the importance of certain fungi has only recently been recognized. The fungi include bodies called mycorrhizas, which are attached to plant roots. The fungi decompose organic matter and incorporate the products in their mycelium. The minerals and organic nutrients are then passed on to the plant roots through the mycorrhizas. As F. W. Went of the University of Nevada has pointed out, this process may be particularly important in badly leached tropical soils, where plant growth depends on the recycling of nutrients from dead to living organic matter and where the principal role of the soil is simply to support the vertical structure of the plants. Other soil microorganisms manufacture antibiotics and growth-promoting organic compounds such as beta-indoleacetic acid and the gibberellins. Went has found that in arid regions the surface layers of sandy soils are held together by microscopic fungi, which stop wind erosion.

In the human food system the prevention of food losses from spoilage is critically important. In the rich countries there is enough energy available to prevent spoilage by refrigeration; in the poor countries less expensive methods must be sought. Among the most widely used are various processes of fermentation by microorganisms, which yield edible and nutritious foods that can be kept until they are needed. The fermen-

	1970			2000		
	CULTIVATED AREA (MILLIONS OF HECTARES)	POPULATION (MILLIONS)	CULTIVATED AREA PER PERSON (HECTARES)	POTENTIAL GROSS CROPPED AREA (MILLIONS OF HECTARES)	PROJECTED POPULATION (MILLIONS)	POTENTIAL GROSS CROPPED AREA (HECTARES PER PERSON)
AFRICA	165	345	.48	995	750	1.33
ASIA	475	2,055	.23	1,100	4,090	.27
AUSTRALIA, NEW ZEALAND	20	20	1.00	125	35	3.57
EUROPE	150	460	.33	245	580	.42
NORTH AMERICA	240	320	.75	695	530	1.31
SOUTH AMERICA	80	190	.43	715	440	1.63
U.S.S.R.	230	245	.94	355	340	1.04
TOTAL	1,360	3,635	.37 (AVERAGE)	4,230	6,765	.62 (AVERAGE)

AMOUNT OF CULTIVATED LAND PER PERSON could be increased in every part of the world between now and the year 2000. Of the 1,360 million hectares under actual cultivation in 1970, only a tiny fraction yielded more than one crop a year. The potential gross cropped area of 4,230 million hectares projected for A.D. 2000 represents a figure that could be achieved by growing more than one crop a year on roughly a third of some 2,900 million net arable hectares. Asia will be hard pressed to obtain the projected ratio of gross cropped area per person. Africa and South America currently offer the largest opportunities for expansion of agricultural production.

tation process not only adds distinctive flavors, which are prized in their own right, but also often augments the content of riboflavin or other vitamins. Sauerkraut and yogurt are familiar fermentation products in American diets; tempeh, ragi, sufu, shoyu, ang-kak, tea fungus and mizo are among those eaten in Asian countries.

More than a century ago Charles Darwin pointed out the important role of earthworms in aerating and turning over the soil. He estimated that an inch of subsoil is brought to the surface by earthworms every five years. Since Darwin's time not much attention has been paid to the valuable activities of worms and other small animals in the soil. One observer in Nigeria has found that earthworm casts corresponding to a layer of soil nearly a centimeter thick were laid down in the course of a six-month growing season.

Almost everywhere in the world the modernization of agriculture will require a large capital investment. In many areas dams, barrages, canals and watercourses need to be built to store, divert and distribute river waters for irrigation. Elsewhere large wells with motorized pumps can be built to tap underground reservoirs that are charged by rainfall and runoff. Whether or not irrigation is needed, farmlands should be properly drained, and that often requires land grading and the construction of drainage channels or underground drains. Most villages in developing countries need farm-to-market roads for bringing in fertilizer and other farm inputs and for transporting harvests. Productivity per hectare will usually increase if farmlands can be leveled or graded, and in many places flood-protecting levees should be built. Large numbers of vermin- and moistureproof structures for crop storage, and also better markets, are needed in most developing countries. Specialized farms for multiplying the seeds of high-yielding crop varieties must be established.

Most of the required capital facilities can be constructed in densely populated poor countries by human labor, with little modern machinery; in the process much rural unemployment and underemployment can be alleviated. On the other hand, heavy investment in machinery and materials will be required for the manufacture of chemical fertilizers, pesticides and farm machinery. During the next 25 years some 400 nitrogen fertilizer plants, each capable of producing 1,000 tons of ammonia per day (or a corresponding quantity of urea) will be needed. The total cost will be at least $40 billion. In 1967 the panel on the world food supply of President Johnson's Science Advisory Committee estimated that doubling agricultural production on currently cultivated land in Asia, Africa and Latin America would require the construction of pesticide plants costing more than $1 billion. In current dollars the cost would probably be twice as high.

In the tropical and subtropical areas where most of the developing countries are located the climate makes possible growing two or three crops a year (wherever enough water can be provided and the soils are not too severely leached). Besides greatly increasing food production such multiple cropping will also increase and stabilize employment. Annual double or triple cropping will be feasible, however, only if the time required to cultivate the fields between harvesting one crop and planting another can be reduced. In order to speed up plowing and cultivating, the traction power now supplied by farm animals may have to be supplemented by small tractors. If crops are to be harvested during the rainy season, mechanical dryers will also be needed. Experience in Pakistan, India and elsewhere shows that such farm machinery, together with motors, pumps and casings for wells, can be constructed by small machine shops in rural towns, using steel and other metals produced in centralized mills.

In traditional agriculture each village is largely self-sufficient, and its social institutions, although often unjust and discriminatory, have been forged by the experience of centuries. New institutions are needed for modern agriculture: banks that can provide loans at relatively low interest rates and that the farmers can invest their savings in, farm cooperatives for the purchase and distribution of agricultural inputs and the marketing of farm products, land-tenure systems that will provide security of tenure to tenant farmers and debt-ridden smallholders, agricultural-extension systems to help in the adoption of new technologies, government price policies that will provide incentives for farmers to increase their production, mechanisms for the distribution and sale of consumer goods to provide farmers with additional incentives, easily accessible and well-staffed schools that will teach the farm children to read, write and do arithmetic, and communications systems between the cities and the countryside that will help to break the crust of custom.

In traditional agricultural societies grinding human labor and simple inherited skills are the principal social factors of production. These societies can be thought of as partly closed ecosystems in which most of the energy derived by people and animals from the photosynthetic product of plants is utilized to grow and prepare food, which in turn provides an essential energy input to grow more food, and so on in an endless cycle. The ecosystems are being disrupted by rapid population growth. I have estimated that in rural India about 40 percent of the food energy contained in the diets of men, women and children over 10 years old is expended to maintain the food system. One of the purposes of agricultural modernization should be to relieve this human drudgery or, in economic terms, to reduce the importance of human labor as a factor in agricultural production.

TYPE OF INVESTMENT	COST (BILLIONS OF DOLLARS)
INCREASE TUBE-WELL CAPACITY BY ONE MILLION CUBIC FEET PER SECOND	3.75
CANALS AND SURFACE RESERVOIRS	16.50
ELECTRIFICATION FOR WELLS	4.50
LAND LEVELING, GRADING, DRAINING	7.50
FERTILIZER PLANTS (5.5 MILLION TONS OF NITROGEN PER YEAR)	1.80
FLOOD CONTROL AND MAJOR DRAINS	5.00
RESEARCH AND EXTENSION; FACTORIES FOR TOOLS, MACHINERY AND PESTICIDES; MARKETING AND STORAGE FACILITIES	2.50
TOTAL	46.55

LARGE CAPITAL INVESTMENTS will be needed for a major increase in crop yield in favorable regions. The table itemizes the investment that would be required to optimize agricultural production on 50 million hectares in India. In order to feed the projected world population of A.D. 2000 many multiples of investment on this scale must be made in Asia, Africa and South America to transform potentially arable land into highly productive farms capable of yielding two or more crops a year. Total cost of this modernization could exceed $700 billion.

One way to accomplish this is to increase scientific knowledge of plant and animal biology and of the environment of water and soils, and to transform scientific advances into practical knowledge farmers can use. The world system of agricultural research institutions is a powerful mechanism for accomplishing both of these tasks. It needs, however, to be supplemented by a large increase in basic biological research. Agricultural biology could well be on the threshhold of a major revolution, based on the new techniques of recombinant genetics, in which genes of diverse species are hybridized, and of somatic-cell genetics, in which single cells are manipulated in special cultures.

Virginia E. Walbot of Washington University has described the dramatic possibilities of recombinant and somatic-cell genetics. In present-day crop-breeding programs the selection of useful characteristics such as pest resistance or high growth rate at subnormal temperatures calls for the raising of tens of thousands of whole plants. At least one growing season is required for finding the desired genetic strain, followed by several more years for finding the seed stock. In somatic-cell genetics millions of cells can be kept in a single test tube, and the generation time is measured in hours or days rather than in months or years. Resistant cells can be selected in a single generation; selected cells can then be cloned to create large numbers of like individuals in a few weeks. It is already possible to regenerate reproductively competent plants from selected cells or from small tissue clumps in approximately a dozen species, including carrots, tobacco and corn. Within the next few decades it should be possible to introduce specific genetic materials into a cereal cell that would determine seed protein content and composition, photosynthetic efficiency, the partition of the photosynthetic product between edible seed and the rest of the plant, and the ability to fix nitrogen.

One of the important discoveries of recent years is that different crop plants have different photosynthetic mechanisms for fixing carbon. The photosynthesis of rice and wheat makes molecules with three carbon atoms, whereas that of maize and sorghum makes molecules with four carbon atoms; the former are called C_3 plants and the latter C_4. C_4 plants exhibit higher photosynthetic efficiency and lower photorespiration, that is, they are able to absorb and utilize more sunlight while losing less of the product of photosynthesis to oxidation during the daylight hours. The C_4 plants do particularly well at higher temperatures; the C_3 plants seem better adapted to lower temperatures. Many native desert species have evolved a third system for taking up atmospheric carbon dioxide at night; it is known as crassulacean acid metabolism (CAM) from the fact that it was discovered and studied in the Crassulaceae, a family of fleshy herbs. Through this mechanism the plants are able to drastically reduce water losses during the daytime.

It may be possible through genetic manipulation to combine the characteristics of the CAM and the C_4 systems, or to combine rice or wheat characteristics with the higher photosynthetic efficiency of C_4 plants. By the year 2000 completely new crop species may have been created by applied genetic research. An ideal new crop species would produce the edible portion of the plant with a photosynthetic efficiency two or three times higher than that of any existing food grain; it would fix its own nitrogen, preferably in the leaves rather than in the roots; the protein in the edible portion would have the balance of amino acids needed by human beings, and the plant would be water-saving, that is, it would evapotranspire much less water per unit of edible product than present-day cereals. It would look and taste, however, like a present-day cereal, and it would be equally capable of being made into bread or pasta or chapati. (We have learned that people are very conservative in their food habits.)

As the foregoing example indicates, many of the factors of production in agriculture are, or could be, interchangeable. The hypothetical new cereal species would require less cultivated land, less irrigation water and less chemical nitrogen fertilizer than any existing food crop to produce the same energy content in edible substance. Nevertheless, because of the dispersed nature of solar energy, the small fraction of sunlight captured in photosynthesis and the need of all plants to evapotranspire water, arable, well-watered land would still be needed.

The physiological requirement for food energy of the average human being is less than 2,500 kilocalories per day, or roughly the quantity of food energy contained in 700 grams of wheat, rice or corn. In the U.S. Midwest the average harvest of corn per hectare is usually more than 240 bushels, or more than 6,000 kilograms, of edible substance. This corresponds to about 60,000 kilocalories of food energy per hectare per day. In other words, 24 human beings can be fed from one hectare of high-quality farmland worked at a level of agricultural technology comparable to that practiced in the U.S. Midwest.

By extrapolation, other things being equal, the present world population of four billion could be fed from 170 million hectares. Yet for the world as a whole at present nearly 1.4 billion hectares are cultivated to provide food, fiber and other agricultural products. There is one hectare of farmland for every 2.9 living persons. There are several reasons for the actual cultivated land per person being eight times the calculated minimum. The land actually harvested during any particular year is about half to two-thirds of the total cultivated land; the remainder is temporarily fallow or is in temporary meadows for mowing or pasture. When chemical fertilizers are not applied, much farmland must lie fallow for a year or more to recover its fertility.

About 10 percent of the cropped area is devoted to raising such nonfood crops as cotton, tobacco, rubber, coffee, tea and jute. Another large fraction is devoted to producing food for livestock and poultry. Some of the livestock provide mechanical energy for cultivating the farms; the products from the rest, including butter, eggs, milk and meat, are eaten by human beings. Livestock and poultry consume from five to 10 times as much food energy as the energy contained in their edible products. From 10 to 20 percent of all food grown is destroyed by pests; a smaller fraction is required for seed.

The principal reason, of course, that so much more land than the hypothetical minimum of 170 million hectares must be cultivated is the low level of crop yields in most of the world. Instead of six metric tons per cropped hectare the average Indian or Pakistani farmer harvests only a little more than a ton of wheat or rice per hectare. A large part of the world's currently cultivated land is less suitable for agriculture than the rich, deep, flat and easily tillable soils of the U.S. Midwest. More important, the level of agricultural technology in the developing countries, which account for more than half of the cultivated land, is very low.

The importance of climate and soil characteristics is illustrated by the differences in the farm value of crops in the 48 contiguous states of the U.S. In Illinois and Iowa that value is more than $130 per hectare of the state's total area; in Delaware and Ohio it is between $75 and $80; in Wisconsin, Mississippi, South Carolina, Georgia and Tennessee it is between $35 and $45, and in West Virginia, Montana, New Hampshire, Utah, New Mexico, Wyoming and Nevada it is less than $10. Nearly twice as much land is cultivated in Kansas as in Indiana, but the total value of the crops is higher in Indiana. The same number of hectares are harvested in Minnesota as in North Dakota, but the crop value is 70 percent greater in Minnesota. On the other hand, the highest dollar yields per hectare of cultivated land (between $1,470 and $1,700) are obtained in Florida, California, Massachusetts and Arizona, four states that differ greatly in soil types, climate and crops. Oranges, grapefruit, tomatoes and sugarcane are Florida's principal cash crops; California grows grapes, hay, tomatoes and lettuce; Massachusetts produces cranberries, hay, tobacco and apples, and Arizona cotton, lettuce, hay and wheat. It is evident that with proper management, sufficient capital investment and satisfactory markets high-yielding agriculture can be achieved over much of the U.S. in spite of the wide range of climates and soil types.

The land surface of the earth outside the ice-covered areas of Antarctica and Greenland has an area of 13 billion hectares. Of this total 2.6 billion hectares are nonarable because temperatures are below freezing in nine or more months of the year. In an additional 1.9 billion hectares there are fewer than three months of the year when available moisture, either from rain and snow or from water stored in the soil, equals or exceeds the potential evapotranspiration from plants and the soil, and there are no practical sources of irrigation water. Climate alone, therefore, limits the area of potentially arable land to 8.5 billion hectares.

The panel on the world food supply of the President's Science Advisory Committee concluded after an intensive study in 1967 that only about 3.2 billion hectares of the total 13 billion hectares of the earth's ice-free land surface can be cultivated. The limitations are due both to climate and to the physical characteristics of the land surface. The panel divided the soils of the world into 13 broad geographic groups. In six of these groups, accounting for 75 percent of the earth's land area, most of the land is not suitable for cultivation. The largest area of nonarable land, 2.6 million hectares, lies in mountainous or arid regions, where the ground is rocky or covered with stony and shallow lithosols. Noncultivable desert soils cover 1.7 billion hectares. The highly leached, acid, dominantly sandy podzol soils in the forested regions of the cool Temperate Zone account for 1.6 billion hectares of nonarable land. Another .7 billion hectares of sandy, undifferentiated soils called regosols are nonarable, and the entire .5 billion hectares of the Arctic tundra are too cold for crops.

Next to the mountainous or arid rocky regions, including the group of lithosols, the largest geographic area is covered by latosols: the reddish or yellowish brown lateritic soils of the savannas and forests of tropical and subtropical regions. These are the most severely weathered and leached soils in the world. Many of them are low not only in phosphorus but also in all the other mineral nutrients necessary for plant growth: potash, lime, magnesia, sulfates and nitrogen compounds. The extreme form of the latosol is laterite, a soil high in iron oxide that hardens irreversibly when it is dried and exposed to the air. Nonarable latosols cover 1.4 billion hectares, yet the latosols also include the largest area of arable land, more than a billion hectares. For high-yielding agriculture, however, these soils must be extensively treated with various supplements, including lime to reduce acidity, and trace metals.

The highest concentrations of arable land lie in the semiarid, subhumid and humid grasslands of the middle latitudes. These are the wheat-producing chernozem soils and the corn-producing brunizems, covering .5 billion arable hectares. Next in quality are the alluvial soils of great river valleys throughout the world, with .3 billion hectares, either actually or potentially arable, and the .2 billion arable hectares in the heavy black grumosols and reddish terra rossas, which are respectively the weathering products of basic and calcareous rocks in warm or hot climates with a well-defined, seasonal rainfall. About a fifth of the area of desert soils and a sixth of the area of podzol soils are arable, and together they provide .75 billion hectares. All other soil groups account for .4 billion arable hectares.

The 3.2 billion arable hectares cover 24 percent of the land area of the earth, about 2.3 times the currently cultivated area and more than three times the area actually harvested in any given year. Of this total .3 billion hectares require irrigation for even one crop.

Irrigation agriculture represents man's principal deliberate use of water, but at present it takes little of the available supply. Slightly more than 1,000 cubic kilometers, less than 4 percent of the total river flow, now irrigates 160 million hectares, which represents about 12 percent of the land area under cultivation. About 10 times 1,000 cubic kilometers of water in the form of rain and snow is evaporated and transpired each year from the remaining 1.2 billion hectares of the earth's cultivated lands and helps to grow food and fiber. Most river waters flow to the sea almost unused by man, and more than half of the water evaporating from the continents, particularly the fraction of the evaporation taking place in the wet rain forests and semihumid savannas of the Tropics, plays little part in human life.

The potential for irrigation development is thus very large, but it is limited by the uneven distribution of river runoff between the different continents and within different climatic zones on each continent. Harold A. Thomas, Jr., Peter Rogers and I have estimated that South America, with less than 15 percent of the earth's land area, accounts for a third of the runoff, whereas Africa, with 23 percent of the land, accounts for only 12 percent of the runoff. Runoff from Southwest Asia, North Africa, Mexico, the U.S. Southwest, temperate South America and Australia accounts for less than 5 percent of the total, yet these regions represent 25 percent of the total land area.

As a result of the uneven distribution of runoff only a third of the land that is potentially arable with irrigation can actually be irrigated (reducing the total potentially arable land to three billion hectares), and the potential increase of the gross cropped area (that is, the sum of potentially arable areas multiplied by the number of four-month-growing-season crops that could be raised in each area) through irrigation development is limited to 1.1 billion hectares. Without irrigation three crops could be grown on .5 billion hectares in the humid Tropics and two crops on .8 billion hectares in subhumid regions. One crop could be grown without irrigation on 1.5 billion hectares. Hence the potential gross cropped area without irrigation is 4.6 billion hectares and with irrigation is 5.7 billion. Of this total, however, 1.5 billion hectares lies in the humid Tropics— where, except for the island of Java and a few other areas with deep, recently weathered soils, no technology is currently available for high-yielding agriculture on a large scale. The potential gross cropped area accessible to relatively high-yielding cultivation with present technology is therefore somewhat more than 4.2 billion hectares [see illustration on page 116].

About 10 percent of the gross cropped area would continue to be needed to grow fibers, beverages and other nonfood crops, leaving a total of 3.8 billion gross cropped hectares outside the humid Tropics for human food production in the future. Making the conservative assumption that lower-quality soils and uneven topography would limit the average yields to half those obtained in the U.S. Midwest, 11.4 billion tons of food grains or their equivalent in food energy could be grown on this potential gross cropped area, enough for a minimum diet of 2,500 kilocalories per day for nearly 40 billion people (if pest losses and nonfood uses could be kept to 10 percent of the harvest).

Besides arable lands, an additional 3.6 billion hectares of the earth's surface could serve for grazing livestock, with an annual animal production of from 25 to 50 million live-weight metric tons. This could provide an average of a few grams of animal protein per person per day for the expected world population at the end of the 20th century.

Because their climates allow growing two or more crops a year over vast regions, the largest potential gross cropped areas are in the developing countries of Asia, Africa and Latin America, which could harvest crops from gross cultivated areas outside the humid Tropics of 1,100, 995 and 715 million hectares respectively. Realization of this potential would require development of irrigation for more than 700 million gross cultivated hectares in addition to modernization of old irrigation systems. It would also require soil supplements for leached acid soils and extensive use of chemical fertilizer to avoid the necessity of fallowing for nitrogen accumulation on more than 1,500 million gross cultivated hectares.

The North American continent ranks just below South America in potential gross cultivated area, with 695 million hectares. The smallest potentials for expansion are in Australia and New Zealand, Europe and the U.S.S.R. In spite of its enormous size, 17 percent of the entire land of the globe, the U.S.S.R. contains only 355 million hectares, or 8.4 percent of the world's potential gross cultivated area. Sixty-five percent of this potential is already cultivated, in contrast to 11 percent in South America and 17 percent in Africa. A large fraction of the potential gross cropped area is also cultivated in Europe (61 percent) and in Asia (43 percent).

Population densities on cultivated land are highest today in Asia and Europe, with .23 and .33 hectare per person respectively, and lowest in Australia and New Zealand, with an average of one hectare per person [*see illustration on page 117*]. The U.S.S.R. cultivates .94 hectare per person and North America .75 hectare. Africa and South America are intermediate, with .48 and .43 hectare per person respectively. If all potential gross cropped hectares could be put under the plow by the year 2000, the harvested area per person would increase on every continent, but only marginally in Asia, Europe and the U.S.S.R. It would increase about threefold in Australia, New Zealand, South America and Africa.

It is obvious that many resources besides arable land and water must be utilized to increase world food production. To realize the earth's full production potential all resources must be available in adequate quantities. Otherwise, in accordance with Justus von Liebig's famous law of the minimum, one resource will be limiting. Some abundant resources can be substituted for scarce ones, but there is no substitute for phosphorus in plant and animal metabolism. It is therefore an essential component of fertilizers for agriculture. Most of the phosphates in fertilizers are ultimately removed from the land and lost in human and animal wastes. Consequently many people have been concerned about the adequacy of future phosphate supplies.

In 1968, 7.6 million tons of phosphorus went into fertilizer. To feed the expected world population of between six and seven billion in the year 2000 it may be necessary to raise the annual application of phosphorus in fertilizer to between 30 and 40 million tons. With current agricultural technology an increase of farm yields by 100 percent would require an increase of 270 percent in the tonnage of fertilizer.

Potential recovery of phosphorus from the known reserves of high-grade phosphate rock has been estimated at 18,000 million metric tons. At the expected rate of application by the beginning of the 21st century, those reserves would be used up in 450 to 600 years. Additional reserves of lower-grade phosphate rock are known to exist. These have been estimated by mining engineers to contain about eight times the amount of phosphorus in the deposits that are economically minable today. Phosphate of still lower concentration is found in many different countries. With foreseeable technology, however, the higher costs of extracting the phosphorus from low-grade deposits would cause a sharp rise in the cost of phosphate fertilizers and hence in the cost of food. Eventually it may be less expensive to recover all the phosphorus that is now removed from the soil in crops and in animal products, and to recycle it for food production.

A large capital investment will be necessary to realize the potential for irrigation and high-yielding agriculture in the developing countries. Cost estimates for the development of 50 million gross irrigated hectares in India are shown in the table on page 118. Even in this ancient cultivated land, where much of the social infrastructure is already in place, the required investment would be close to $1,000 per hectare. Making the highly uncertain assumption that costs elsewhere in Asia, Latin America and Africa would be the same as in India, a total of more than $700 billion would be needed for irrigation development and agricultural modernization on these three continents, including the cost of adding lime and other soil supplements to the severely leached latosols. If this investment were spread over 25 years, the annual cost would be $30 billion, less than 1 percent of the present gross world product. Because of the shortage of capital in the developing countries, a large part of this investment would need to come from the developed countries. It would seem to be a small price for the transformation in the lives of the world's poor (probably one of the necessary conditions for reducing birthrates) that could be brought about by the modernization of agriculture.

11

The Amplification of
Agricultural Production

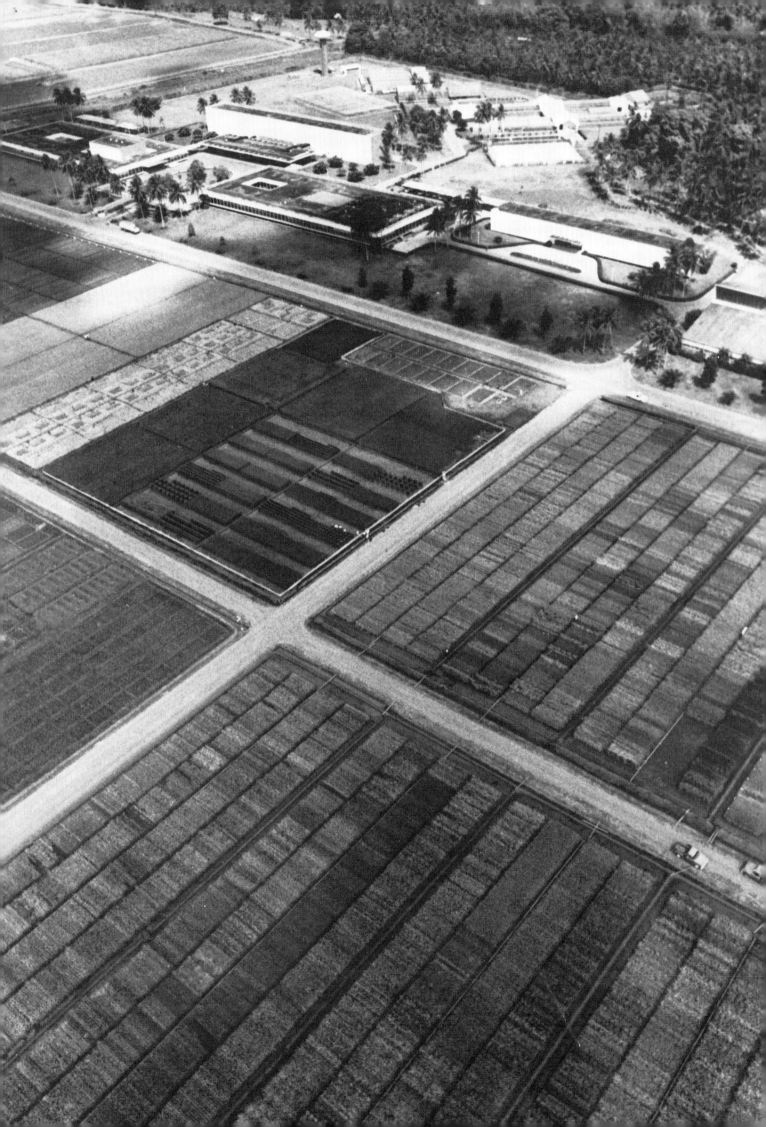

The Amplification of Agricultural Production

PETER R. JENNINGS

The new technology of the green revolution brings larger harvests from a given area of farmland. The foundation of this technology is the breeding of crops adapted to the needs of intensive agriculture.

The modern rebuttal to the Malthusian prophecy is the potential of agricultural technology for greater yields, that is, for growing more food on each acre of land under cultivation. Some remarkable gains in productivity have been achieved. The first large-scale successes came in the 1920's and 1930's in the developed countries of the Temperate Zone. In the developing countries of the Tropics and sub-Tropics, where the need for higher yields is now the most urgent, a comprehensive program for increasing farm productivity has only recently been established. It has already made substantial progress with at least a few crops, notably wheat and rice. The early successes of the program earned it the name "green revolution."

The central element in the endeavor to improve yield is the breeding of new varieties of crop plants. A first imperative is the development of varieties that produce abundantly when they are grown in dense plantings and are supplied with fertilizer, water and pesticides. The plants can also be given other desirable properties, such as resistance to diseases and to insects and tolerance of a wide range of climates, soils and other environmental factors. In principle every heritable characteristic of the plant is subject to the will of the plant breeder.

Recent increases in wheat and rice production in a number of developing countries testify to the potential power of plant-breeding programs. Even for wheat and rice, however, the quest for improved crops is by no means finished, nor can it ever be truly finished, and there are many other crops in the developing world that demand equal attention. The green revolution did not solve the problem of world food supply; rather, it demonstrated an approach to a solution, a method. That method can be successful only if it is applied continuously to crop improvement.

Plant breeding has a long heritage in those parts of the world that are today considered less developed: all the major food crops were domesticated there. The farmers of the Neolithic period were adept at observing variations in plant populations, selecting the seed of the better specimens and replanting the outstanding varieties. Constant selection pressure was applied over thousands of years, and the plants that survived and reproduced were those favored by man. Progress was not rapid, but the total contribution of the ancient agriculturists rivals that of modern professional plant breeders.

In the process of domestication, species with great native variability were introduced into innumerable environments, and the types that performed best in each area were perpetuated. Thousands of distinct varieties were created, each one well adapted to some limited area. Many of those varieties have survived; for example, more than 30,000 kinds of rice have been collected. The multitude of existing varieties is of incalculable value today. Early peoples in the Tropics were largely responsible for the creation and preservation of what has become the greatest resource of modern plant breeding: abundant crop germ plasm.

The breeding methods devised by Neolithic man remained standard until the 20th century, although in recent decades they were applied more systematically and with more sophistication. The technique is called pure-line selection. The breeder begins with a mixed population of plants and selects the seed of those that appear to have the characteristics he wants. The seed is grown, and from the progeny the best seed is again selected. Through explicit tests of the pure-bred lines, such as exposure to drought or to predation by a particular insect, the most tolerant or resistant varieties can be selected. When applied with diligence and careful observation, pure-line selection can result in considerable improvement. The fundamental limitation of the method is that it exploits only those genetic combinations that are found in nature. If a desirable trait is discovered, it can be utilized only in the variety that happens to possess it, which may have undesirable traits as well. The pure-line method offers no way of transferring a trait from one line to another.

The modern era of plant breeding began at the turn of the century with the rediscovery of the laws of inheritance formulated by Gregor Mendel in the 1860's. Those laws hold that inheritance proceeds through the assortment of distinct and discrete traits determined by genes. The genes behave as units that segregate during reproduction and are randomly redistributed in all possible combinations in the offspring. The laws of inheritance imply the possibility of creating new combinations of genes, and hence varieties not seen in nature.

The basis of a modern breeding program is cross-pollination, or hybridization. For naturally self-pollinated crops,

HIGH-YIELDING RICE in experimental plots at the International Rice Research Institute (IRRI) at Los Baños in the Philippines appears in the aerial photograph on the opposite page. IRRI was the first in a network of international institutes established to improve the yield of crops in the developing countries. The essential element in this program was the development of dwarf varieties of the cereal crops, including rice, that would respond to applied fertilizer. Large numbers of plants are crossbred, and the resulting genetic types are evaluated for their potential yield and for many other characteristics. A measure of the genetic diversity of the crop is suggested by pattern in these fields: each stripe represents a breeding selection of rice.

such as wheat or rice, the procedure begins with two purebred lines, each of which has traits considered valuable. The two lines are cross-pollinated and the resulting seeds are grown, the hybrid progeny being termed the F_1 generation.

All the plants in the F_1 generation are identical, but when they are inbred by self-pollination, a great range of diversity appears in the next generation, which is designated F_2. The F_2 generation contains an enormous number of new genotypes: all the possible combinations of the parental traits are represented. Those that have inherited the desirable characteristics of the parental varieties are selected, and by repeated self-pollination additional generations are grown (designated F_3, F_4 and so on). With each generation additional selections are made, eliminating the less desirable genotypes. As the inbreeding continues, the population becomes more stable, and by about the F_6 generation the selected lines are essentially true-breeding. Beginning with the F_2 generation the plants are evaluated individually for disease resistance, height, quality and many other properties, and the selections are guided by the results. Eventually field trials of the true-breeding lines are undertaken in various environments. The end result is the selection of a single genotype representing the optimum combination of the parental characteristics.

There are a number of variations on the basic hybridization procedure that are available to the plant breeder. For example, additional genetic material can be introduced into a line by crossing a third parental variety with an F_1 hybrid, or by crossing two different F_1 hybrids. There are also a number of limitations, the chief one being that in certain cases genes for different traits are linked: they are close to one another on a single chromosome and therefore tend to be inherited as a unit. On the whole, however, crop germ plasm has considerable plasticity, and with persistence and sufficient resources a plant variety with most of the desired characteristics can be developed.

Plant breeding is largely a matter of numbers: the more lines hybridized and the more plants grown from each hybridization, the greater the chance of finding outstanding specimens among the progeny. In recent years breeding programs in the Tropics have become very large. Hundreds of hybrids are produced each year and from them tens of thousands of breeding lines are established; millions of individual plants are grown and evaluated. Moreover, in the tropical environment it is possible to grow two or three generations a year under diverse conditions. Breeding projects in the U.S. tend to be much smaller. The tropical programs work with a larger volume of experimental material, and they produce finished varieties faster.

The native, unimproved varieties of crops such as wheat, rice and maize are not inferior per se. Given the conditions under which they have been grown, they may represent the optimum choice from among the available varieties. Moreover, the farmers who have grown them for generations are neither backward nor incompetent; on the contrary, their practices reflect a sound agricultural and economic strategy.

In traditional agriculture the fertility of the soil is often the factor that limits growth. Nitrogen in particular is commonly in short supply, and the shortage is severer in tropical soils than elsewhere. The native crop varieties extract nitrogen and other nutrients from the soil with great efficiency. They develop extensive root systems, drawing on a large area of soil, and they exhibit vigorous growth, which suppresses weeds that compete for the available nutrients. Having been bred by traditional methods of selection for thousands of years, they have acquired a precise, although narrow, adaptation to the local conditions, including peculiarities of the soil, the water supply, the length of the growing season, average and extreme temperatures and the photoperiod, or number of daylight hours, which is a function of latitude.

A native variety of a crop is rarely a purebred line; instead it is a population in which all the members may have similar outward characteristics but have varied genotypes. Populations of this kind are called land races. The genetic diversity of the land race can be of great value to the traditional farmer, since it confers at least partial resistance to insect predation and disease, and partial tolerance of environmental stresses such as drought. If a crop becomes infected with a particular disease, for example, some of the strains in the land race are

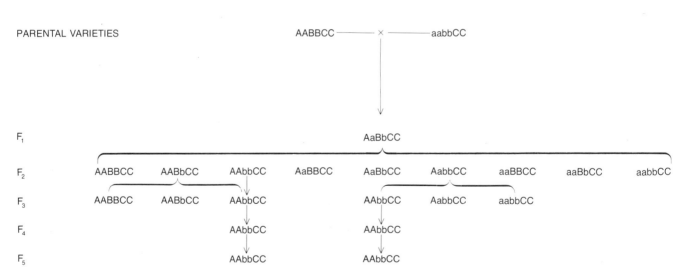

PARENTAL VARIETIES

AABBCC ——————— × ——————— aabbCC

F_1 AaBbCC

F_2 AABBCC   AABbCC   AAbbCC   AaBBCC   AaBbCC   AabbCC   aaBBCC   aaBbCC   aabbCC

F_3 AABBCC   AABbCC   AAbbCC   AAbbCC   AabbCC   aabbCC

F_4 AAbbCC   AAbbCC

F_5 AAbbCC   AAbbCC

CREATION OF HYBRIDS and selection from among their offspring are the basic techniques in the development of new crop varieties. With rice the process begins with the cross-pollination of two purebred lines of plants. Here the plants are shown as having genes for just three traits (A, B and C), and each gene is assumed to have only two forms (represented by uppercase and lowercase letters). The progeny of the cross-pollinated plants are designated the F_1 generation; all these plants are identical and all of them have an equal share of genes from each parental line. The plants of the F_1 generation reproduce by self-pollination, and in their offspring (the F_2 generation) a great range of genetic diversity appears. Here, where the parental varieties differ in only two traits (A and B), the F_2 generation has nine distinct genotypes; crop plants ordinarily differ in many more traits, and large numbers of plants must be grown in order to sample the multitude of possible genetic combinations. In the F_2 generation the plant breeder can begin to select plants by saving the seed of those that possess more desirable characteristics. In succeeding generations the selection is intensified, and the population becomes more stable as more and more plants are genetically uniform. Through hybridization the best characteristics of many plant types can be incorporated into a single variety. Here the genotype $AAbbCC$, which did not appear in either one of the parental rice varieties, has been selected.

likely to be susceptible, but others may well be resistant and will survive. Moreover, the nonuniformity of the plant population tends to limit the maximum numbers of pests and disease organisms and thereby to prevent disastrous crop failures. The net effect of this agricultural system is to give the farmer a measure of security. The strategy of the subsistence farmer in particular is not to obtain the greatest yield in the best of years; instead he must ensure some yield even in the worst years.

The main failing of the traditional agricultural system is that yields cannot be significantly increased. The one reliable way to obtain more crop per hectare is to grow more plants per hectare, which obviously requires that the plants be placed closer together. With the unimproved types that is not possible because of their characteristic large size and because they compete strongly for light and nutrients. Moreover, the land could not sustain the additional population of a denser planting. The nutrient pool of the soil would quickly be exhausted and the plants would not receive enough sunlight; as a result they would not develop properly.

The solution to the problem of nutrient depletion is chemical fertilization, including a generous nitrogen supplement; that is the only way to sustain the higher plant density required for higher yield. When a native variety is grown with a large dose of fertilizer, however, several new problems emerge. First, most of the newly available nutrients are employed not for increasing the edible portion of the plant but for vegetative growth. Leaf area increases greatly, and because the plants are closely spaced each one shades its neighbors; as a result the overall photosynthetic efficiency of the crop is reduced. With cereal crops an even more serious problem arises. Because fertilization increases the size of the plants in traditional varieties, the grain is borne on a much-elongated stalk. Long before the grain is ripe it has become too heavy for the straw, and in wind or rain it "lodges": the straw bends or breaks and the grain falls to the ground, where much of it is lost.

The problem of lodging and of excessive vegetative growth has been solved by breeding dwarf and semidwarf varieties of the major grains. Indeed, the development of these varieties is the very heart of the green revolution. The dwarf plants have short, upright leaves, so that in dense populations the plants do not shade one another. Their straw is also short and stiff, and capable of supporting a full head of grain to maturity. The root systems are relatively small, but extensive root systems are not required because fertilization ensures an adequate supply of nutrients. Fertilizer is an essential in the cultivation of the new

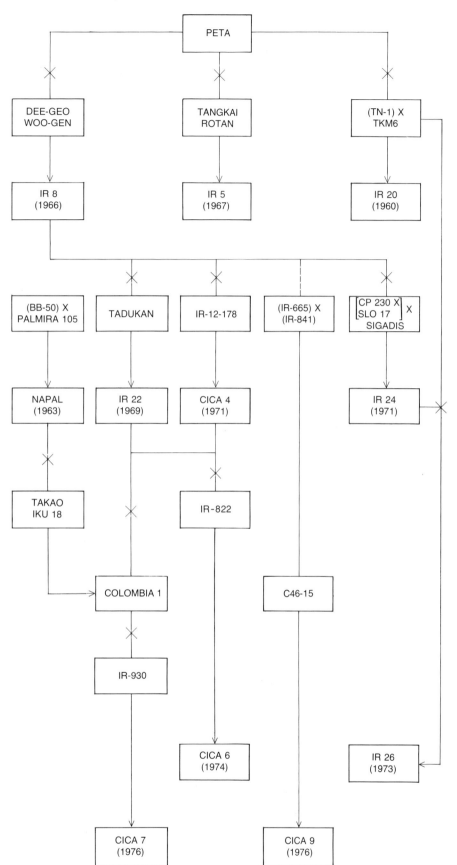

GENEALOGY of selected modern rice varieties maps a complex sequence of hybridizations. Most of the modern varieties are dwarf or semidwarf plants that can be planted in dense populations and heavily fertilized to attain high yields. Those whose names begin with the letters IR were developed by IRRI; those with the letters CICA were developed by a collaboration of national and international agencies in Colombia. The first of the modern types to be widely adopted was IR 8; it was created by crossing Peta, a tall Indonesian rice known for vigorous growth and other desirable properties, with *Dee-geo woo-gen*, a dwarf variety from Taiwan.

varieties; without it they do no better than the traditional types, and they may do worse. Although some of the varieties have a broad resistance to diseases and pests, chemical pesticides are frequently applied, and management of weeds and the water supply is also necessary. These requirements add to the cost of growing a crop, but the investment is amply repaid by the increase in productivity.

The transformation of tropical agriculture began in Mexico in 1943, in a cooperative project sponsored by the Rockefeller Foundation and the government of Mexico. The goal of the project was to increase production of the basic food crops in Mexico, and initially much emphasis was placed on improving spring wheat. The methods and the mode of organization employed in this early program have strongly influenced the subsequent course of development elsewhere.

A small staff was assembled, consisting mainly of Mexican nationals and in-

cluding specialists in several disciplines (plant breeding, plant pathology, soils, entomology and farm management) and communications specialists who would serve as intermediaries between the research station and operating farms. A simple and pragmatic goal was set: to quickly obtain a large increase in national wheat production. All other concerns were subordinated to this goal. An important feature of the Mexican program was the formation of interdisciplinary teams in which each member contributes expertise in his own field. This approach to agricultural research differs from that of most institutions in the U.S., where plant breeders are often isolated from their colleagues in related fields. In Mexico the emphasis on interdisciplinary teams was to a large extent responsible for the success of the program, and the same plan of organization has been adopted by most other crop-improvement programs in the Tropics.

The Mexican wheat team immediately set about collecting genetic resources. Lines of wheat were acquired from all

regions of the Western Hemisphere and from East Africa, the Middle East and South Asia. Crosses between these lines and native Mexican wheats were screened for yield, for insect and disease resistance and for range of adaptation, particularly with regard to photoperiod and temperature. The critical lodging problem was solved in 1953 with the successful crossing of Mexican varieties and North American semidwarf wheats. The dwarf genes in the American types were derived in turn from a group of Japanese semidwarf types called Norin. When the first semidwarf varieties were introduced, productivity had already been substantially improved; the short-statured wheats brought an additional large increase in yield.

In the 1940's Mexico had been importing half of the wheat it consumed in order to make up a deficit in production; yields averaged 750 kilograms per hectare. By 1956 the nation was self-sufficient in wheat in spite of a large increase in population. By 1970 yields had reached 3,200 kilograms per hectare.

From the start of the wheat-improvement project the screening of experimental varieties included field tests overseas, in which the improved Mexican selections were crossed with local varieties. By the mid-1960's the success of this program had been demonstrated, largely because of the broad environmental adaptation of the varieties. Beginning in 1966 seed was exported in quantity, mostly to India, Pakistan and Turkey. Record harvests were achieved almost immediately.

The second great triumph of tropical plant breeding came with rice, after the establishment in 1960 of the International Rice Research Institute (IRRI) in the Philippines. The approach taken was similar to the one that had proved successful in Mexico. Again international and interdisciplinary research teams were assembled, and again a pragmatic goal of improving yield on the farm was given the highest priority. Germ plasm was acquired from all the rice-growing nations of the world; the institute's collection now contains more than 30,000 varieties. It was soon recognized that the first requirement would be a short-statured rice that could be planted in dense populations, that would resist lodging and that would respond to heavy fertilization by increasing the production of grain rather than foliage.

It is worth considering in some detail the procedures and problems involved in such a breeding program. Both rice and wheat are naturally self-pollinating, and hybridization is a delicate and time-consuming procedure. Each floret on the plant must be opened and the pollen-bearing anthers removed before they mature. Later, anthers from the chosen parental variety are broken over the

RESPONSE TO FERTILIZER is the most important factor contributing to improved yields of cereal crops. The response is markedly different for IR 8 (color), a modern dwarf variety, and Peta, a tall traditional type. In the absence of nitrogenous fertilizer Peta may be superior to IR 8, but the yield of both varieties is low. When Peta is heavily fertilized, however, it becomes too tall, and the stalk can no longer support the head of grain. The plant is then subject to "lodging": the stalk bends or breaks and the grain falls to the ground, greatly reducing the effective yield. IR 8 has a short, stiff stalk capable of holding the grain aloft until it is harvested.

stigma in each floret, and the entire flower cluster is enclosed in a bag to protect it from stray pollen.

The resulting hybrid seed, which yields the F_1 generation, is generally grown under protected conditions, but the F_2 and later generations go to several outdoor nurseries and to greenhouses where the plants are exposed to controlled stress. In the F_3 and later generations the performance of all selections is determined in the field under standard conditions, for comparison with that of other lines, and the range of adaptation of the plants may be checked by evaluation in other parts of the world. If a particular trait is being sought, such as resistance to a known virus, then a series of test screenings, involving several generations, is undertaken. The results of any of these procedures may indicate the need for further genetic manipulation. Finally, a successful experimental variety must be grown in farmers' fields in a variety of geographic and climatic regimes, and its performance must be analyzed both agriculturally and economically. Because the development process is elaborate and because many generations of rice must be grown to maturity, the creation of a new variety requires several growing seasons.

The first improved dwarf varieties of rice were released by IRRI in 1966; they immediately transformed rice culture in the Philippines and were soon widely adopted in the lowland regions of Asia. One variety in particular, designated IR 8, gained widespread celebrity. It has the potential for high yield when properly fertilized and cultivated, it is insensitive to photoperiod and it is adapted to a broad range of growing conditions. Moreover, it matures in 120 days instead of the 160 days required for many unimproved types. Because of the earlier maturity two crops a year can be grown in some regions.

More recent varieties developed by IRRI and several national research programs incorporate other desirable traits. It had become obvious early in the history of the program that disease resistance is of paramount importance: the fields of the institute itself were decimated by plant viruses. Some recent lines combine resistance to several of the bacterial, viral and fungal diseases of rice and to the insects that both damage plants directly and serve as vectors of the viruses. The discovery of parental stock resistant to these pests and diseases requires mass screening of 10,000 or more varieties, followed by hybridization to incorporate the resistance genes into improved types. Lines have been established that are tolerant of drought and of adverse soil conditions. Ongoing programs match the characteristics of the grain to the preferences of consumers and increase the protein content of the grain. Finally, in a few varieties the growing season has been reduced to 100 days, which in some irrigated regions makes triple cropping feasible.

When the Mexican wheat-improvement program was established, a parallel program to increase yields of maize was also begun. Maize is grown widely by subsistence farmers in Latin America, and also in Africa and in some parts of Asia. Yields have traditionally been low.

It was in maize that the methods of 20th-century plant breeding were first successful in the developed countries, and particularly in the U.S. The important contribution was a method for the commercial production of hybrid maize, which was devised in the 1920's and 1930's; by 1950 hybrids had been almost universally adopted in the U.S. corn belt. Yields increased roughly fivefold in less than 20 years.

For farmers in the developing nations the cultivation of hybrid maize does not appear to be practical. The hybrids grown are of the F_1 generation, and all the plants in a given population are genetically uniform. Such uniformity increases the vulnerability of the crop to diseases and insects, and in the Tropics those stresses are particularly severe. Hybrid maize has another disadvantage: for F_1 hybrids new seed must be produced each year by the deliberate crossing of carefully maintained purebred lines. The developing countries lack the facilities for producing the seed or for distributing it, and subsistence farmers may not be able to afford the recurrent cost of seed. The traditional practice since Neolithic times has been to save a portion of the harvest as seed for the next crop.

Methods for breeding maize are different from those for wheat or rice. Maize bears separate male and female flowers, as opposed to the perfect flowers of most cereal crops, and under natural conditions it is almost always cross-pollinated. Lines that are deliberately inbred soon become weak and stunted. The hybrid varieties grown in the U.S. were developed explicitly to counteract this tendency, but the maize-development program in Mexico has placed little emphasis on the creation of hybrids. Instead populations of plants have been developed that are in effect land races composed of much-improved individuals. The plants in a given population are similar in appearance and are uniform in properties such as length of growing season, but they are genetically diverse. The plants are grown and pollinated by natural methods for several generations, with only the seed of the favored individuals saved at each harvest. In this way the frequency of desirable genes in the population gradually increases, although a given gene is not likely to be present in every plant. Deliberate cross-breeding is still a basic element in the improvement program, but the object is merely to incorporate new traits into the heterogeneous population, not to create a purebred variety.

As in the breeding of wheat and rice,

VARIETY	STATURE	DISEASE RESISTANCE				INSECT RESISTANCE			GROWING SEASON
		BLAST FUNGUS	BACTERIAL BLIGHT	GRASSY STUNT VIRUS	TUNGRO VIRUS	GREEN LEAF-HOPPER	BROWN PLANT HOPPER	STEM BORER	
IR 8	DWARF								120 DAYS
IR 20	DWARF								120 DAYS
IR 26	DWARF								120 DAYS
IR 28	DWARF								105 DAYS

□ RESISTANT
□ MODERATELY RESISTANT
▨ MODERATELY SUSCEPTIBLE
■ SUSCEPTIBLE

DESIRABLE PROPERTIES incorporated into rice varieties through the breeding programs at IRRI and other institutions include short stature, which has a direct effect on yield; resistance to diseases and insect pests, and a short growing season. IR 28, a variety released in 1974, has broad disease and pest resistance and a growing season shorter than that of most traditional varieties. Because of the earlier maturity some farmers can grow two crops a year or even three. Other characteristics that are shared by some or all of the new rice varieties include insensitivity to photoperiod (the number of hours of daylight) and tolerance to inhospitable soils.

a first objective in the maize-improvement program was the breeding of plants that could be grown in dense plantings and that could be fertilized without danger of lodging. This was accomplished by literally shifting the center of gravity of the plant: crossbreeding tall, tropical plants with dwarf varieties has produced a shorter plant that bears the ear of grain lower on the stalk. The improved populations also have shorter leaves, and the leaves remain upright. Genes that confer resistance to disease and insects have been bred into some of the better populations. As a result of these changes it has been possible to increase the crop density from 50,000 plants per hectare to more than 100,000.

For many years it appeared that broadly adapted varieties of maize could not be created. Instead separate populations were developed for various altitudes, latitudes and growing seasons. Since about 1970, however, some populations with a fairly wide range of adaptation have been created. Sensitivity to photoperiod, for example, has been reduced by crossbreeding selected varieties from different latitudes. In some cases broad-spectrum disease resistance has also been achieved.

Progress in maize improvement has not been as rapid as that in wheat and rice, but it has not been negligible. In Mexico productivity has doubled, and the technology has been exported to Africa and Asia.

The results of the programs outlined above must be considered encouraging, but one should remember that they concern only three crops and that they have reached only limited areas of the world. Continued progress can be achieved only through continued research directed toward eliminating constraints on productivity.

Ralph W. Cummings of the Rockefeller Foundation recently published a survey of the state of food-crop technology in the low-income countries. He compared the average annual gain in production for 15 basic commodities during two periods, 1961 through 1965 and 1971 through 1973. His findings give a rough indication of the contribution of research to food production since World War II. Two conclusions emerge from the study. First, an evaluation of the status of research on the major food crops indicates that in almost all cases research is "seriously inadequate" or "critically inadequate." Only the specialized areas of irrigated rice and irrigated spring wheat were considered to have received adequate research attention. Second, annual gains in production of seven crops (cassava, white potato, soybeans, cowpeas, broad beans, maize and wheat) were greater than 2.5 percent, and thus equaled or exceeded the rate of population growth. Most of those gains, however, resulted from increases in the area under cultivation. Although exceptions were noted in some countries, for the most part the increases in production could be attributed to higher yields—and hence to agricultural research—for only two crops: irrigated rice and irrigated wheat. The remaining crops in the survey—sorghum, pigeon peas, dry beans, chick-peas, ground nuts, sweet potatoes and millets—failed to keep up with population growth in both total production and productivity.

The prospects for immediate improvement in the national agricultural research programs of the developing countries are not encouraging. Salaries and research funds are inadequate, and few who are qualified are attracted to careers in agriculture. Many who start in agricultural research turn elsewhere for better salaries, weakening the leadership and continuity of the programs. Unfortunately the growing need for trained plant breeders in the developing countries coincides with a decline in the practicality of plant-breeding instruction available in the developed nations. In the U.S., for example, publicly supported plant breeders, as opposed to geneticists, are becoming rare, and excellence in postgraduate training in applied breeding is to be found at only a few institutions. Specialized research in genetics will someday contribute to varietal development and to higher farm productivity, but in the meantime traditional fieldwork in plant breeding must not be allowed to deteriorate.

A new threat to the well-being of crop research is the attitude of those who, rightly impressed by the advances of the past decade, have come to believe that there is a surplus of useful knowledge and that all that remains is to deliver the new varieties and cultural practices to the farmers. Some concerned with the allocation of resources in the developing countries have advocated a shift in financial support from research to extension services. That position is unrealis-

INSTITUTE	AREAS OF RESEARCH	FUNDED	LOCATION
INTERNATIONAL RICE RESEARCH INSTITUTE (IRRI)	RICE	1960	PHILIPPINES
INTERNATIONAL MAIZE AND WHEAT IMPROVEMENT CENTER (CIMMYT)	WHEAT, MAIZE, BARLEY, TRITICALE	1966	MEXICO
INTERNATIONAL INSTITUTE OF TROPICAL AGRICULTURE (IITA)	CORN, RICE, COWPEAS, SOYBEANS, LIMA BEANS, ROOT AND TUBER CROPS	1968	NIGERIA
INTERNATIONAL CENTER OF TROPICAL AGRICULTURE (CIAT)	FIELD BEANS, CASSAVA, RICE, CORN, FORAGES, BEEF PRODUCTION	1969	COLOMBIA
INTERNATIONAL POTATO CENTER (CIP)	POTATOES	1972	PERU
INTERNATIONAL CROPS RESEARCH INSTITUTE FOR THE SEMI-ARID TROPICS (ICRISAT)	SORGHUM, MILLETS, CHICK-PEAS, PIGEON PEAS, GROUNDNUTS	1972	INDIA
INTERNATIONAL LABORATORY FOR RESEARCH ON ANIMAL DISEASES (ILRAD)	LIVESTOCK DISEASES	1973	KENYA
INTERNATIONAL LIVESTOCK CENTRE FOR AFRICA (ILCA)	AFRICAN LIVESTOCK	1974	ETHIOPIA
INTERNATIONAL CENTRE FOR AGRICULTURAL RESEARCH IN DRY AREAS (ICARDA)	WHEAT, BARLEY, LENTILS, BROAD BEANS, OILSEEDS, COTTON	(PLANNED)	LEBANON

AGRICULTURAL RESEARCH in the developing countries is conducted by a network of international institutes in cooperation with national research programs. Each of the institutes is concerned with particular crops (or livestock), and some of them confine their interest to a particular region or climatic regime. All the crop research institutes employ an interdisciplinary approach in which plant breeders, plant pathologists, entomologists, economists and others work together to improve the productivity of crops in farmers' fields. Since 1971 the institutes have been funded in large measure by the Consultative Group on International Agricultural Research (CGIAR), which is an association of national governments, specialized agencies of the United Nations and private philanthropic foundations.

tic. As we have seen, most of the crops of the Tropics have not yet approached their potential yield. Even after productivity goals have been attained crop research must go on. An established variety of a crop plant exists in continuous coevolution with the organisms that compete with it and prey on it, and resistance cannot be maintained indefinitely. In tropical agriculture the pressures of disease, insects and weeds are intense, and new varieties remain useful only about half as long as they do in the Temperate Zone. Plant breeders must work that much harder to keep up.

In spite of these portents I believe that recent developments in agricultural research give reason for optimism. By far the most important factor is the creation of a new network of international agricultural institutes that work closely with national research programs. IRRI, founded in 1960 and initially supported by the Ford Foundation and the Rockefeller Foundation, was the first of these institutes. The second was formed in Mexico in 1966 when the wheat- and maize-improvement programs begun in the 1940's were consolidated in the International Maize and Wheat Improvement Center, or CIMMYT (from the Spanish name Centro Internacional de Mejoramiento de Maiz y Trigo). CIMMYT too was initially funded by the Ford and the Rockefeller foundations, which also helped to establish an International Institute of Tropical Agriculture (IITA) in Nigeria and an International Center of Tropical Agriculture (CIAT) in Colombia. In 1971 the financial support of these organizations was assumed by a consortium of donors organized as the Consultative Group on International Agricultural Research (CGIAR). The sponsors of the CGIAR are the World Bank, the Food and Agriculture Organization of the United Nations and the United Nations Development Program, but several nations and private philanthropic foundations are also members. The CGIAR has funded four more institutes, including two concerned with livestock, and an additional crops research institute is planned. In 1976 the eight existing institutes have been pledged $65 million by the member governments and agencies of the CGIAR.

The research programs of the international institutes are organized on a pattern that is now familiar. Teams of young career investigators representing several disciplines are brought together to work on a common problem. Their objectives are simple and pragmatic: to identify the factors that most severely limit yield and to alter them in such a way as to increase production. Each of the institutes has a limited sphere of interest, confined either to a region or to a particular crop or group of related

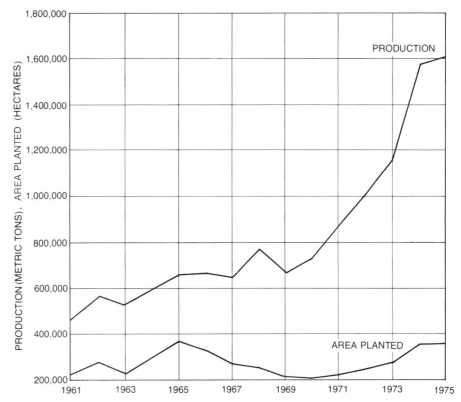

RICE PRODUCTION in Colombia rose sharply following the introduction of improved dwarf varieties in the late 1960's. The varieties were developed jointly by the International Center of Tropical Agriculture (CIAT), the rice-improvement program of the Colombian government and the Colombian National Rice Growers' Federation. The dwarf lines were first planted in 1968, and by 1974 they were being cultivated on virtually all of the land in Colombia that was sown to irrigated rice. By 1975 the annual production had increased by almost a million metric tons over the rate that had prevailed before the breeding program went into operation.

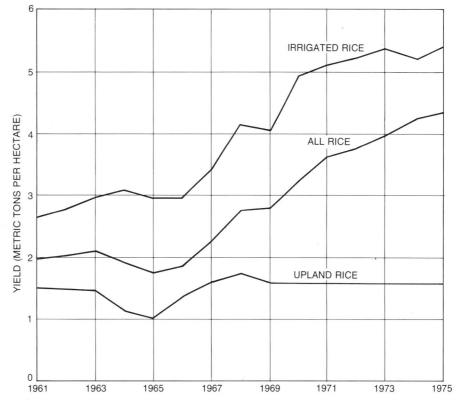

INCREASED YIELD of Colombian rice is almost entirely responsible for the increase in production. That the improvement in yield was brought about by the adoption of improved varieties is suggested by the fact that only irrigated rice is affected. Upland rice varieties, which are grown without irrigation, were not included in the country's rice-improvement project.

crops. New technology is evaluated on farms in many countries, ensuring broad applicability and encouraging the participation of national agricultural agencies. Finally, through the routine work of the institutes scientists from the national research programs are trained in the methods and materials of practical plant research.

The concept of the multinational, interdisciplinary research team in agriculture may ultimately prove to be the most significant contribution of the institutes. The need for plant-breeding teams is critical in the humid Tropics, where the biological constraints on farm productivity are diverse and severe. The international teams not only have made direct contributions through the institutes but also have helped to revitalize some national research programs. Hundreds of investigators, working at experiment stations in their own countries after training six months to a year at one of the institutes, form a corps of production-oriented workers around whom national research programs are growing. They evaluate the findings of the institutes in their own countries, modify them as needed and form a direct link between the institutes and the farmers.

The early successes of the green-revolution crops were exhilarating because they demonstrated the enormous potential of tropical agriculture. There have been a few more demonstrations of the power of technology to transform both the land and the people who live on the land; one of them involves the growing of irrigated rice in Latin America.

The rice varieties developed by IRRI have been widely adopted in Asia, but they require further adaptation before they can be planted in other parts of the world. In 1967, in an effort to extend the new methodology to Latin America, an IRRI rice breeder was transferred to CIAT in Colombia. At the same time several Colombian workers were sent to IRRI in the Philippines and elsewhere for academic and practical training in aspects of production research. A comprehensive regional breeding program was established jointly by CIAT and the Colombian government in collaboration with the Colombian National Rice Growers' Federation. Liaison with national research programs in other Latin-American countries was established by training more than 90 foreign nationals in Colombia, who returned to their own countries to evaluate the latest plant-breeding materials and cultural practices under the conditions that were prevailing there.

The collaboration of an international institute, a national research program and an organization representing producers developed technological "packages" that were tested directly on farms. Several new dwarf varieties were released by the program in Colombia, and others were developed in other countries from material distributed by the Colombian project.

The program was successful not only in the development of new rices with a potential for high yields but also in introducing the new varieties into the national agricultural system and actually achieving those yields. In Colombia the first plantings of improved rice were made in 1968. By 1974 more than 99 percent of the land area growing irrigat-

COSTS AND BENEFITS of the Colombian rice-improvement program clearly justify the expenditures necessary for agricultural research. The costs of research led to small deficits until 1967, but the value of the additional crops harvested had paid for the entire program a few years after the improved varieties were introduced. In 1974 the additional annual production was valued at $230 million, compared with a research expenditure of $340,000. Most of the benefits of the program were passed on to consumers in the form of lower prices for rice. The graph is based on a study of the program by Grant M. Scobie and Rafael Posada of CIAT.

ed rice was planted to one of the improved dwarf lines.

The impact of the new technology is readily measured. Yield has risen from less than three metric tons per hectare to 5.4 metric tons, so that each hectare planted to the new varieties produces 2.5 metric tons of additional grain. Total production increased from 680,000 metric tons in 1966, the year before the program began, to 1,632,000 metric tons in 1975. Almost all the increase was accounted for by improved yield. The value of the additional crops harvested through 1974 was about $450 million. Varieties derived from the Colombian project were also successful in Mexico, Ecuador, Peru, Venezuela and in Central America. Throughout the region the 1974 harvest was increased by 1.5 million metric tons of grain.

For many of the noncereal crops improvement remains more a matter of manifest potential than of accomplish-

ment. An example is cassava, a root crop known in the U.S. mainly in the granulated form called tapioca, but a dietary staple in many tropical countries. Cassava was largely neglected until CIAT in Colombia and IITA in Nigeria recently undertook to improve it. It has the potential for enormous yields, up to 50 tons per hectare, and grows well even in relatively poor soils. In actual production, however, yields are generally less than 10 tons per hectare.

The technology required for cassava improvement is rapidly being acquired. Breeding teams from the international institutes, in collaboration with national programs, are developing high-yielding varieties and the cultural practices that must accompany them. Yields of from 30 to 40 tons per hectare have been obtained on farms in a wide range of environments. It is a rule of thumb that when farm trials yield from two to three times the national average, there is a potential

for rapid growth in regional production. A remaining need is a technique to reduce storage losses of freshly harvested roots. When that becomes available, cassava production should increase.

The recent transformation of irrigated rice culture in Colombia is a compelling argument for the value of crop research. Indeed, it suggests that the best investment the international community can make in the developing countries is in agricultural research aimed at increasing the productivity of food and other crops. Since 1967 the annual expenditure on rice research and related activities by CIAT, the Colombian government and the Colombian Rice Federation never exceeded $1 million. In Colombia alone and in one year alone, 1974, the added production resulting from the introduction of the new technology was valued at $230 million. That is a splendid return on any investment.

12

The Development of Agriculture
in Developing Countries

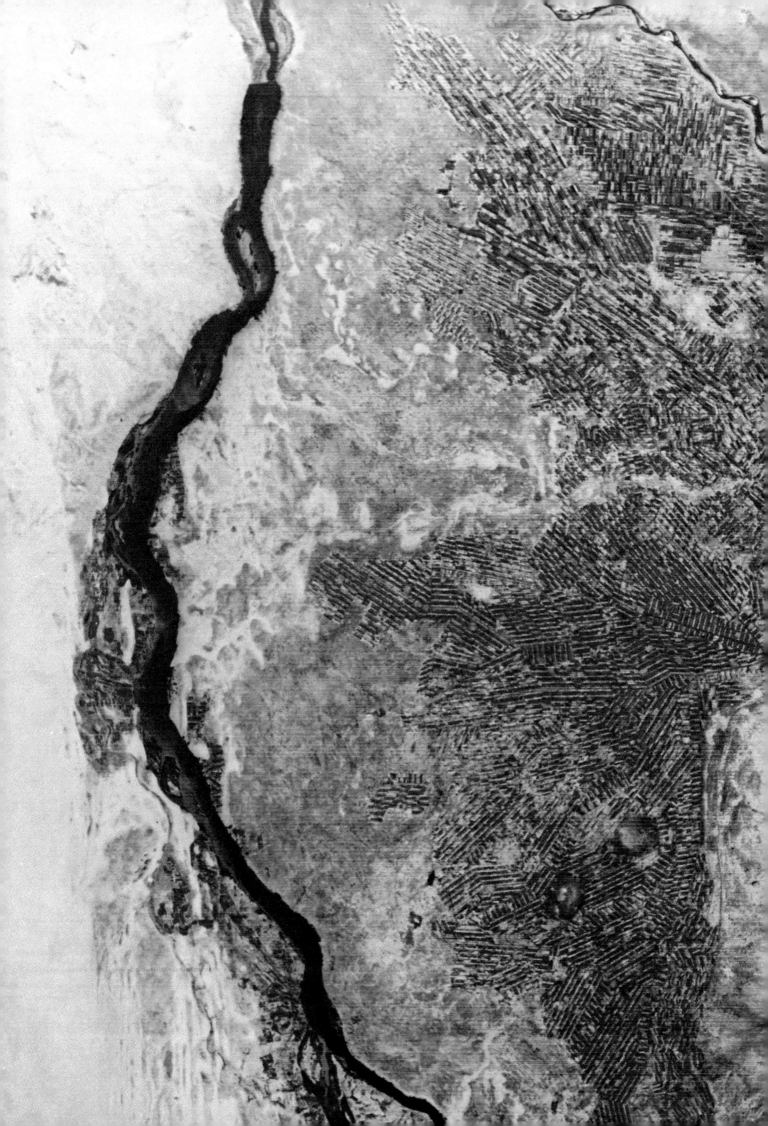

The Development of Agriculture in Developing Countries

W. DAVID HOPPER

The poor countries can feed themselves if their agriculture is modernized and their rural economies are restructured. That requires infusions of technology and capital from rich nations

If the people of the poor countries are to be fed, the food will have to come from their soil, their resources and their farm economies. The surplus production of a few exporting countries can serve on occasion to buffer the impact of bad weather or other calamities, natural or man-made, but there should be no illusion that the world's food security can be ensured by abundant harvests from the fields of Kansas and Saskatchewan, Argentina and New South Wales. Very few of the developing nations give evidence of having understood that food independence is an internal affair, and that if agricultural development is given priority, it can lay the foundation for modernizing an entire economy. The rich industrial nations have also not fully recognized that such development, on which depend both the world's future food supply and an easing of the tension between the rich and the poor, calls for a massive transfer of technology and capital from rich to poor countries.

Alternatives have been suggested, to be sure. One, known euphemistically as the lifeboat analogy, holds that the earth can support only a limited number of people and that those of us who are safely aboard must not jeopardize our ability to survive by extending a helping hand to the billions of others who would

swamp the vessel. A modified version of this ethic is called triage, after the battlefield aid-station practice of categorizing the wounded in three groups: those likely to survive without immediate attention, those likely to die in any case and those who can be saved if they get immediate attention. Under this rule some countries would receive help but the Bangladeshes of the world would be abandoned. Both of these approaches seem to me almost as impractical (dying countries are not as easy to dispose of as drowning people or stretcher cases) as they are indecent.

A third suggestion, infinitely more humane, is based on the fact that rich populations consume about five times as much grain as poor ones because they process most of it into meat—an inefficient conversion. If North Americans were to reduce their bloated diets by about a third, the argument goes, they would make 78 million metric tons of cereal grains available to those who need it. The trouble with this is that the 78-million-ton dividend would be reduced as the American population grows and would soon fall behind the growing populations and rising standards of food consumption in the developing countries; this form of distributive economics cannot for long do

anything but distribute poverty. Moreover, merely saving food does not give anyone the money to acquire that food. Finally, the domestic political and economic obstacles to reducing American meat output make such a program not only ineffective but also unlikely. There is room for distributive justice in the world, but it should take the form of economic assistance, commodity-pricing agreements and trade reforms that give the poor nations a better chance at development.

As I said at the outset, that development should be in the first instance agricultural, something that is hard to impress on most developing-country governments. They tend to prefer such attributes of modernity as national airlines and smoking industrial plants to simple farm-to-market roads, bags of high-yielding wheat seed, rural credit cooperatives and other levers of agricultural transformation. And yet most of the developing countries are better endowed for agricultural progress than for any other kind of economic advance. The developing world lies largely on and between the tropics of Cancer and Capricorn. It is a belt of warm temperatures, of generally abundant (if often seasonal) rainfall and of ample, year-round solar energy to be converted into chemical energy for storage in plant and animal tissue.

The tropical and subtropical resources of the developing countries are now mainly exploited by farming techniques that have remained almost unchanged for centuries. Yields per hectare and per farm worker are very low (which largely accounts not only for the world food shortage but also for the poverty of most of the world's farmers). It is now clear, however, that where modern plant varieties and farming techniques are introduced, farmers succeed in wresting from their land single-crop yields two or three times as large as

IMMENSE POTENTIAL of the developing countries in the tropical and subtropical regions of the world for producing their own food is suggested by the LANDSAT composite image on the opposite page, which shows part of the two-million-acre Gezira irrigation complex in the Sudan. (The area included in this view is roughly 50 percent larger than other full-page LANDSAT scenes in this issue.) The irrigation works here, located in the fertile clay-soil plain between the White Nile and Blue Nile rivers just south of Khartoum, were originally developed in the 1920's by the Sudan Plantation Syndicate, a British-managed venture primarily devoted to growing cotton. Since the works were nationalized more than 25 years ago the emphasis has been shifted to food crops and to more intensive agriculture. In the decade between 1960 and 1970 the proportion of land cropped annually increased from 47 percent to 62 percent; almost half of the increase was accounted for by the introduction of wheat. In this LANDSAT 2 false-color image, recorded on December 7, 1975, the cultivated strips of land appear red and the fallow strips appear green. Farther south in the Sudan the great swamps formed by the White Nile constitute what is potentially one of the richest farming regions in the world, with the soil, sunlight and water resources to produce enormous quantities of food.

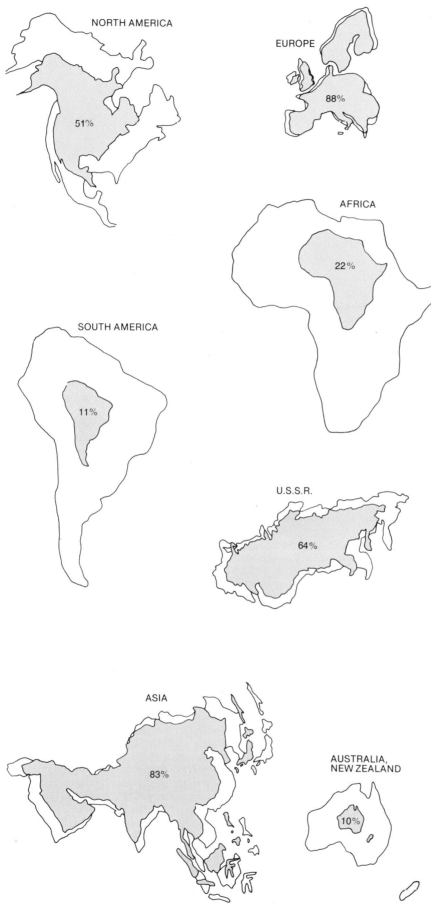

NORTH AMERICA

51%

EUROPE

88%

AFRICA

22%

SOUTH AMERICA

11%

U.S.S.R.

64%

ASIA

83%

AUSTRALIA, NEW ZEALAND

10%

EXPANSION OF FARMING to arable but as yet uncultivated land would be one way to increase the world's food production. The outline maps show the world's major landmasses, sized in proportion to the area of their potentially arable land. The silhouette map (*color*) within each outline shows how much of that potentially arable land was being cultivated as of the mid-1960's. The numbers give the cultivated area as a percent of the potentially arable area.

the traditional return; multiple cropping of two or three crops on the same piece of land—something that is peculiarly feasible in the Tropics and sub-Tropics—gives yields from four to eight times larger than traditional ones. Specialists in agricultural development now believe new farming systems can be specifically designed for various tropical and subtropical conditions that hold immense promise of greatly enhanced output, better year-round utilization of farm labor and a significant opportunity to improve the nutritional and economic well-being of the small cultivator. That is the first step toward not only a new agriculture in the developing countries but also economic health.

The significance of the "green revolution" derives not so much from its numerical impact on food output as from its demonstration of what is involved in the modernizing of traditional agricultures. The widespread, rapid adoption of high-yielding varieties of wheat and rice gave proof that peasant farmers were not slow or stubbornly resistant to change. Aggressive adoption of new farming techniques had a long history where cash crops were concerned, but the myth persisted that because most of the food grown in developing countries is destined for the cultivator's own consumption, traditional production technologies would be slow to change. This was not the case. Within four years of the first widespread release of the seed of new high-yielding wheat varieties in South Asia those varieties occupied practically all the land suited to their cultivation. In response to yield differences of 200 to 300 percent over traditional plant varieties, and with the important incentive of grain prices that made high-yield farming extremely profitable, the Asian peasant proved to be as innovative as any in the world; the stereotype of the traditional farmer, slow to change and stubbornly resistant to progress, died a much-deserved death.

The experience with high-yielding wheat and rice was important on several counts. It was the first time large numbers of farmers had made significant innovations quickly in their food-production methods. It was the first time many developing countries had achieved substantially higher yields of food crops from previously cultivated land through the application of nontraditional technologies derived from scientific research; until then increases in food output had come either from extending cultivation to uncultivated land or from improving land with irrigation facilities. And finally, it provided the first clear evidence that, if new farming technologies do add greatly to yield, if the added yield can return a profit beyond the enhanced cost of the new methods and if farmers have access to the production factors (such as seed, fertilizers and insecticides) and the capital resources (such as irrigation facilities and farm machinery) they need in order to apply these methods effectively, then aggressive innovation will follow.

Subsequent research has identified access to production factors and the expectation of economic returns from innovation as crucial requirements. The high-yielding varieties differed from traditional genetic types in their response to plant nutrients, particularly to nitrogen, which is usually the major limiting factor in the warm soils of the Tropics [see "The Amplification of Agricultural Production," by Peter R. Jennings, page 125]. The farmers' access to supplies of fertilizer was therefore critical in fostering innovation. A large quantity of crop water was also indispensable. High-yielding crops make maximum use of solar energy only when their leaf canopy is dense. A dense plant population absorbs (for photosynthesis, respiration and transpiration) much more water than the thin crop cover of traditional,

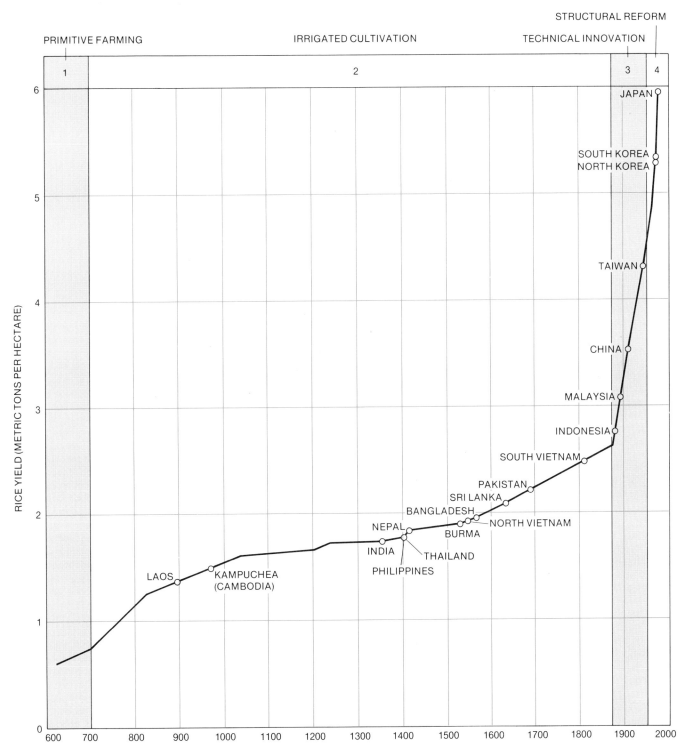

INTENSIFICATION OF FARMING on land now being farmed is the other way to grow more food. This means moving farming in developing regions to higher stages of development, in effect recapitulating the historic progression exemplified here by the case of Japan. Kunio Takase of the Asian Development Bank found that typical rice yields in Japan increased (*black curve*) as Japanese agriculture moved from the traditional stage through the advent of irrigation to scientific agriculture and finally to structural transformation. Current yields in most Asian countries, where less than 50 percent of the rice land is cultivated, place them still in second stage, as plotted.

low-nutrient farming. The farmers who could benefit from adopting the technologies of the green revolution were those within easy reach of depots handling fertilizer supplies and whose fields were either supplied by irrigation systems with abundant water or were located in areas of assured rainfall.

On the economic side modern techniques of food production require purchased inputs, something that was not usual in traditional farming. Although most traditional farmers have had some contact with a cash economy, for many of them the risks of farming, and in particular the vulnerability of the farm family to cash indebtedness arising from a crop failure, put a brake on innovative behavior. This is particularly true for farmers with small landholdings and little accumulated wealth. Unassisted, they are the last to change their practices; they wait until more affluent neighbors have experimented with the new methods, and in many circumstances they avoid risk by not adopting the new ways at all. For them and even for many of their wealthier neighbors the adoption of new agricultural technologies depends not only on the effect on production, possible profit and access to supplies but also on the availability of credit, of risk insurance and of farm-extension advice, which reduces the likelihood that one will unwittingly neglect some important component of what is often a complex package of interlocked farming practices. The need for cash inputs for food farming implies the need for access to product markets, since there must be some way of obtaining money from the sale of crop surpluses to pay for the production factors. Thriving markets depend on transportation networks, storage facilities, processing plants, a system for the dissemination of market information, the availability of credit for traders and so on.

Those are some elements of the infrastructure required for a market-oriented agriculture; some others are complexes of technological research services, economic institutions to support farmer credit and to facilitate trade, extension advisory services for farmers and the industrial base to produce farm inputs. Such institutions and facilities are weak or lacking in developing countries, which is why the way to world food security is also the way to their economic development.

The new dwarf wheat and rice varieties, together with fertilizer and assured water, more than doubled India's wheat output between 1968 and 1972, gave Pakistan an exportable rice surplus and brought the Philippines within striking distance of self-sufficiency in food. The opportunity for profit that those varieties opened to farmers resulted in an unprecedented dynamic of development in the regions suited to their cultivation. Private-farmer investment in irrigation, in land improvement, in modern tillage equipment and in improved storage facilities was a major result of the transition from a traditional basis of food production to a scientific basis.

The green revolution experience contains two broad lessons. The first is the importance of the impact on land areas already under the plow of modern agricultural technologies that are economically rewarding for the cultivator to apply and whose application is capable of being supported by an off-farm infrastructure of the appropriate services. The second is the lack of much interaction between the social and cultural institutions of a society (such as the pattern of land tenure) and technological and economic change. Land-tenure reform has long been held to be a necessary first condition to generating growth in farm output, for example. It is undisputed that very large landholders may, and often do, keep land unfarmed or otherwise fail to maximize its agricultural productivity. In such cases land redistribution or some form of economic incentive or punishment is appropriate in order to make the land productive. In regions that are already cropped or grazed to the limit of traditional technologies, however, farms can benefit from modern methods whether they are large or small. And there is evidence that if they are properly assisted with nonfarm services, all those who work the land will increase their output, regardless of their position on the land-tenure ladder. Judging by the record of the diffusion of the dwarf varieties of crops, it is true that small farmers, having fewer resources, are slower to adopt new methods. Once the new practices have proved to be profitable, however, and assuming that the availability of credit is not a barrier, small farmers can and do become as innovative as larger landholders. This is not to deny that rural institutional reform is vitally necessary in many, if not most, developing countries. Its justification, however, rests primarily on the need for the better distribution of social, economic and political justice; it is only marginally relevant to the expansion of farm output.

In a recent study the International Food Policy Research Institute estimated that in order to avoid a deficit position by 1985 the developing countries must increase their cereal-grain output at a rate of approximately 4.25 percent per year from 1976 on. That is two and a half times the 1.69 percent rate they attained between 1967 and 1974 and more than one and a half times the 2.5 percent rate that was the average for the past 15 years. There are basically two ways of attaining that level of growth in output: by the expansion of farming to land not now being cultivated and by the intensification of production on land already being cultivated.

Large areas of the Tropics are not farmed or grazed, and they constitute a huge reservoir of future production [see "The Resources Available for Agriculture," by Roger Revelle, page 113]. The southern half of the Sudan is potentially one of the richest farming regions in the world, with the soil, sunlight and water resources to produce enormous quantities of food—as much, perhaps, as the entire world now produces! The water is useless today: the headwaters of the White Nile, blocked in their northward flow by high plateaus, spill out over the land to form great swamps. To unlock the promise of the southern Sudan those swamps would have to be drained, a rural infrastructure put in place and the nomadic cattle raisers of the region somehow changed into sedentary farmers. The capital costs of such an undertaking would be as large as the promise, and the time required would cover generations. Yet the potential is real and untapped, and as world food shortages persist such a reserve cannot long be neglected.

The extensive llanos of Latin America—the flat, grassy plains north and south of the Amazon basin—are unexploited tracts that, with a sufficient investment in rural infrastructure, could be made highly productive for ranching. Other areas with an immense potential for adding to human food supplies are the savannas of Africa, the tens of millions of hectares of semihumid land south of the Sahara now closed to human habitation by onchocerciasis, the river-blindness disease, large regions of tropical forest and even some of the desert regions of the Arabian Peninsula, North Africa and western Asia.

Before these reservoirs of future food production can be tapped, research on the farming and development technologies suited to their individual ecologies will have to be undertaken and the political will and political action of nations and the world community at large will have to be mobilized to ensure a sustained flow of development resources. The Sudan, for example, is desperately poor, with a gross national product about equal to the 1974 net income of the International Business Machines Corporation. From this economic base the Sudanese alone cannot possibly subjugate their swamps, harness their rainfall and establish a farm economy on their tremendous land resource.

The second and much greater potential for expanding food production lies in the intensification of farming in areas that are already being cultivated or grazed. The productive capacity of these areas cannot be doubted: they are already supporting almost two-thirds of mankind on a traditional, low-yield technological foundation. If these resources were exploited by modern means, no child would need to know hunger and no people would need to fear famine. For example, if its glacial waters and rainfall were harnessed and its farmers better supported by modern off-farm services, the 40 million hectares of the Indus-Ganges-Brahmaputra plain of Pakistan, Bangladesh and India could be made to yield upward of 20 metric tons of cereal grain per hectare per year, or about 80 percent of the world's present cereal output. The capital cost would be high, perhaps as much as $50 billion over the next 25 or 30 years, but that is about 17 percent of the estimated global expenditure on armaments and military establishments in the single year 1976. These river basins, if developed, alone would meet world food needs for the next 14 years, even allowing for a growth in demand of 4.25 percent per year.

Similar comments can be made about almost every other farming area of the tropical and subtropical developing world. In the South Asian case I have just cited, however, there is the advantage of a fairly highly developed rural economy; the need now is for a large investment in structural transformation so that the entire rural sector can be geared to the demands of a high-productivity agriculture. This structural transformation is the last stage in what has been seen as a four-stage progression in agricultural development. The long first stage is that of traditional farming, with reliance on traditional implements and practices and on rainfall for water. In the second stage the productivity of the land is improved by irrigation and drainage, by the enhancement of soil nutrients through better incorporation of organic materials and by the better timing of crop production through improved implements for cultivation. The third stage is marked by the introduction of scientifically developed techniques. Cultivation of dwarf varieties on irrigated land with purchased fertilizer is a typical development of this stage; another is the introduction of vaccines and dips to control livestock diseases. The fourth stage is the structural transformation of a rural economy, which involves establishing the full range of institutions and infrastructures needed to support a high-productivity agriculture.

The history of Japanese agriculture provides the clearest example of the four stages. Traditional Japanese farming relying on rainfall returned rice yields of less than one metric ton per hectare. The extension of irrigation between A.D. 600 and 1850 raised yields to 2.5 tons. The Meiji restoration in the 1870's ushered in a long period of scientific innovation in which high-yielding

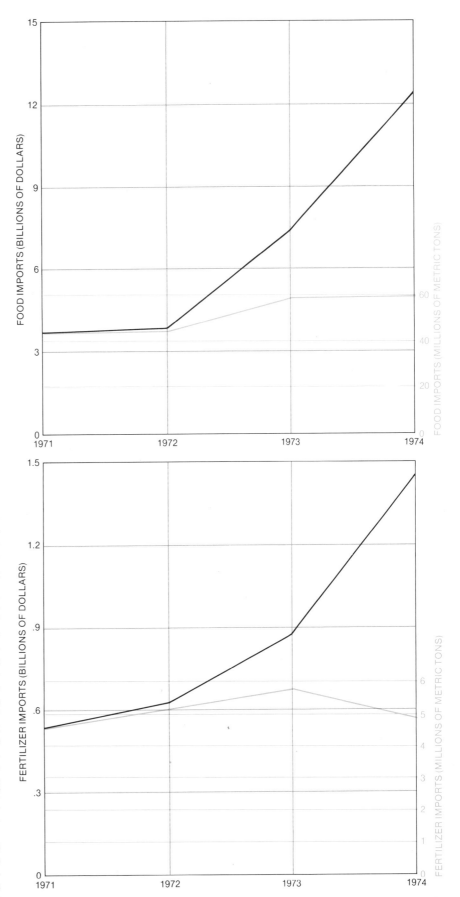

INFLATION has made it harder for developing countries to import the food they need or the inputs required to grow it. The charts show the amount of money (*black curves*) spent in four recent years by developing countries to import food (*top*) and fertilizer (*bottom*), along with the quantities of food or fertilizer (*color*) the money bought. Top chart includes China and oil-exporting developing countries; bottom one does not. Data were compiled by Overseas Development Council from publications of United Nations Food and Agriculture Organization.

varieties, fertilizers and other chemicals, improved implements and better agronomic practices were investigated by scientists, tested by a network of prefecture research stations and then demonstrated to farmers. Between the late 19th century and World War II rice yields rose from 2.5 tons per hectare to four tons. The postwar reorganization of Japan's farmland, the strengthening of farm-supply and marketing industries and trading channels, the establishment of farmer organizations and the opening of more agricultural schools and colleges—in brief, the structural transformation into a complex modern rural economy—pushed rice yields to the present level of almost six tons per hectare, and many observers believe eight tons will be reached in the not too distant future.

In contrast to Japan, most of the other nations of Asia are only now making the transition from the first to the second stage, from traditional farming to an agriculture based on increased land productivity. The extension of irrigation and drainage, essential to high-productivity rice cultivation, is being laboriously pursued in the South Asian and Southeast Asian nations. Except in western Malaysia, where the irrigation potential is well developed, rice yields are still below two tons per hectare. The introduction of scientific production technologies and the new dwarf, high-yielding varieties in these nations has been mainly limited to areas commanded by irrigation; in India and Pakistan about 30 percent of the cropped area is so commanded. Indeed, the present evidence strongly suggests that entry into the stage of successful technological innovation in the developing countries of Asia depends on a prior capital investment in the productivity of the land. That is, the second stage must precede the third.

Most of Africa is still in the first stage of traditional farming. In order to unlock the potential of their soils the African nations, the poorest in the world, must therefore be prepared to make a colossal investment in land productivity, in agricultural scientific research and extension services and in the structural development of their farm economies. Large areas of Africa are and will continue to be mainly devoted to the raising of cattle. The development of watering places, improved ranges, disease-control centers, meat-packing establishments and other facilities could dramatically enlarge Africa's ability to add to world food supplies, particularly to the supply of protein. Africa's potential is suggested by its existing examples of modern farm development. Some of the areas that were settled by European farmers are among the most productive in the world. Their high productivity can be traced to the large investments made in roads, supply depots, markets, farm equipment, research and extension and farmers' organizations, and in the economic institutions and government policies necessary to make all those elements function.

In Latin America, where there is an abundance of unfarmed or traditionally farmed land, the overall problems are not unlike those of Africa. The recent upsurge in Brazilian agriculture, if it is sustained, will soon carry that nation into cereal export markets. If the development plans of Venezuela and Colombia meet with even partial success, those nations should also be net contributors to world food supplies. Chile, Argentina and Peru have large unexploited farm potentials that are currently unfulfilled because of government economic and development policies for rural areas.

If the output from single crops grown on land now being cultivated or grazed through traditional techniques can be multiplied by five or six, as it has been in Japan, or even by two to four, as it has been on the limited-rainfall central plains of North America, present world production would almost double. If the potential for the multiple cropping of the warm Tropics is tapped, global output could climb five or six times above its present level of approximately 1.2 billion metric tons of cereals.

Intensive multiple cropping in the Tropics implies extensive irrigation and mechanical tillage. Supplementary water in the dry seasons is a precondition for wresting from the land two or three crops a year. And the short intervals between crops makes rapid land preparation and careful timing of farm operations a necessity, something that can be accomplished only with modern power sources and implements. The results are dramatic. Single-crop yields can be tripled in the course of a year if planting times are kept short and rapidly maturing varieties are sown. If synergistic crops are interplanted in the rotations so that they overlap from one planting to the next, the output of the land can be raised another 50 to 60 percent. The combined effect—improving single-crop yields in each segment of a multiple-crop rotation—has raised the total output of a hectare of land from a traditional one-crop-per-year level of less than two tons to more than 20 tons. Such results have been attained on carefully controlled experimental plots; ordinary farmers, properly guided, could be expected to increase their present yields between five and seven times.

As one considers the tropical farming world and the technology now available or soon to be available, there can be no grounds for pessimism about the latent potential of the world to feed increasing numbers of people for a long period ahead. Whether that latent potential will be harnessed to the benefit of man is the question. There has been much talk in both the developed and the developing nations about the need to accelerate agricultural development. The need remains, but the required political actions are not being taken.

Part of the blame can be placed on the developing countries themselves. Agricultural development is expensive and other, often more glamorous priorities of modernization shoulder aside its claim for scarce resources. Rural development is also a politically charged endeavor. City dwellers are more clamorous of attention, and their demands are more urgent and visible than those of a traditional peasantry. Keeping food cheap to appease urban consumers often leads to policies that destroy the economic incentive for modernizing farms. And the rich countries are always offering food on easily negotiated concessional terms. The food generosity of the industrial countries, whether in their own self-interest (disposing of food surpluses) or under the mantle of alleged distributive justice, has probably done more to sap the vitality of agricultural development in the developing world than any other single factor. Food aid not only has dulled the political will to develop agriculture but also, by augmenting domestic production with grain grown abroad, has kept local prices at levels that destroy incentives for indigenous farmers. In the last analysis making surplus food cheaply available to the developing countries in normal times has reinforced the already strong tendency of those countries to neglect local agriculture; it is easier on their national budgets to farm the fields of the U.S. and Canada.

Among the large, populous developing nations only China seems to have brought its agricultural development into an approximate balance with demand. China imports wheat and exports rice; the net has recently been on the import side, but since about 1971 China has been essentially self-sufficient in food. Authoritative Chinese data are hard to find, but on the evidence available Chinese agricultural output rose by about 3.4 percent per year between 1960 and 1974. Estimates of population growth in China are even sketchier, but it seems to be between 1.5 and 2 percent per year, and decreasing. If these data are correct, and barring emergencies, the outlook for the Chinese food situation is good.

China has accomplished its agricultural growth largely by mobilizing and disciplining its farm labor. The role of the political cadres in providing leadership and social control in the commune structure is well documented. Personal incentives, work assignments and tight enforcement of social discipline multiply the effectiveness of traditional labor-intensive methods. The Chinese are also emphasizing modern technical inputs, and these will increase markedly in the future as the plan for a very large expansion in fertilizer capacity is met.

The Chinese experience rests on the Maoist philosophy that the way to communism in China is through its rural masses, not through the heavy industrial development of the Russian model. China, unlike most other developing countries, has given pride of place in its development to the transformation of traditional farming. Whether China's methods of effecting the transformation are applicable to other societies and other cultures is a debatable question; the unique characteristics of Chinese culture may be more important for China's rural success than any particular techniques for accomplishing political and social change. Other countries, notably Tanzania, are experimenting with forms of social development that adapt many features of the Chinese model to their circumstances. It is too early to pass judgment on these activities, but they are worth watching for the lessons to be learned.

Food aid aside, the record of the developed nations is no better than that of most of the developing ones. As a group the rich nations have been devoting decreasing proportions of their gross product to official development assistance for developing nations. An inadequate percentage of that aid goes for agricultural and other rural purposes: in 1974 it was about 23 percent, or a little more than $2.6 billion, an amount far below the need. Moreover, much of that is accounted for by what is called technical assistance, which means paying one's own nationals to work in developing countries. That does not provide capital, which is what the poor countries need above all.

The 1974 World Food Conference was given a figure of $5 billion a year for the next 20 to 25 years as a conservative estimate of the foreign exchange needed by the developing countries for investment in food production if the world is to attain a secure annual food supply. To mobilize such resources the conference called for the creation of three new international bodies: the World Food Council, the Consultative

Group on Food Production and Investment and the International Fund for Agricultural Development (IFAD). Since the conference in 1974 there has been some progress. The council, a body of representatives from ministries of agriculture in 36 nations, has met twice since 1974 to review efforts being made to implement the global development of agriculture and food-producing capacity. The consultative group is striving to coordinate worldwide investment in agriculture. IFAD was formally agreed to in June, with an initial subscription of close to $1 billion by the Western industrial countries and the members of the Organization of Petroleum Exporting Countries (OPEC). This year the Arab countries established an Arab Authority for Agricultural Investment and Development with an initial capitalization of $525 million and a six-year plan for investing $2.8 billion in rural development and food production in the Middle East, with particular attention to developing the resources of the southern Sudan. The various agencies of the World Bank have given increasing priority to agriculture and rural development, doubling their support for those categories

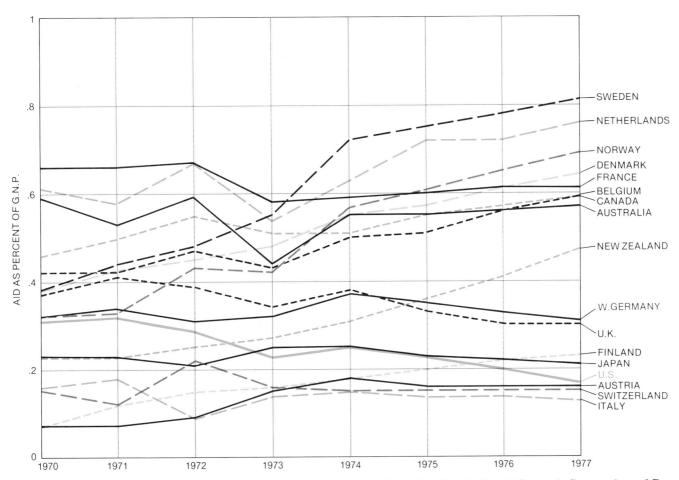

DEVELOPED COUNTRIES are now devoting a smaller proportion of their output to official development assistance than they were in the mid-1960's. The curves show such aid as a percent of gross national product for member countries of the Development Assistance Committee of the Organisation for Economic Co-operation and Development. The UN target for official development assistance is .7 percent of G.N.P. Disbursements were projected to 1977 by World Bank on the basis of national policy statements and appropriations.

in 1975 compared with the previous year.

Even if it is considered narrowly in terms of eventual payoff, capital devoted to agricultural technology and infrastructure is well invested. Irrigation offers a good example. A long-term global approach to food security must rest on the development of water resources and the widespread extension of modern irrigation technologies. Nowhere is this better demonstrated than in Israel, where farm output has grown some eightfold in the past 25 years, largely through the efficient utilization of water. Modern water-resource development and the accompanying irrigation and drainage works are capital-intensive and expensive. A recent investigation sponsored by the French Ministry of Cooperation has found that even the rivers and groundwater of the semiarid Sahelian zone of Africa, the scene of a recent devastating drought and famine,

could be harnessed over the next 75 years to provide crop water for almost 2.5 million hectares, at a cost likely to be in excess of $25,000 per hectare. The return on such an investment is hard to calculate, but a conservative estimate of yield would be 10 tons of cereals per hectare per year, or an output of about $1,500 per hectare: a 6 percent gross return. That is a minimum return, since it is likely that land of such value would be planted to crops with a higher economic return than cereals provide.

The relevant question for mankind, however, may not be one about investment return. It may rather be: What is the long-run cost of not initiating now a program of investing in man's future food supply? Water-resource development has a long gestation time before it yields benefits, and so do many other elements of agricultural modernization. Political leaders in both the rich and the

poor countries have a short time horizon; they focus on immediate concerns. Yet future food supplies depend not on the application of more fertilizer to existing fields this year or next but on a joint and shared commitment by the developed and the developing countries to the long-term and expensive development of the world's untapped farm resources.

It is important to recognize that the world's food problem does not arise from any physical limitation on potential output or any danger of unduly stressing the "environment." The limitations on abundance are to be found in the social and political structures of nations and in the economic relations among them. The unexploited global food resource is there, between Cancer and Capricorn. The successful husbandry of that resource depends on the will and the actions of men.

The Authors
Bibliographies
Index

The Authors

STERLING WORTMAN ("Food and Agriculture") is a vice-president of the Rockefeller Foundation. A plant geneticist by training, he holds degrees from Oklahoma State University and the University of Minnesota. Since joining the staff of the foundation in 1950 he has worked as a corn breeder in Mexico, a pineapple breeder in Hawaii and a rice breeder in the Philippines. He has been based at the foundation's New York headquarters since 1966, when he became director of its agricultural-sciences division; he took up his present job four years later. Wortman currently serves as president of the International Agricultural Development Service and as a member of numerous boards and committees, including three for the National Academy of Sciences: the Board on Science and Technology for International Development, the Committee on Scholarly Communication with the People's Republic of China and the Steering Committee of the President's Study on Food and Nutrition. In past years he has been a trustee of the International Rice Research Institute in the Philippines, vice-chairman of the board of trustees of the International Maize and Wheat Improvement Center in Mexico and a member of the World Bank Advisory Panel on Agriculture and Rural Development. Among his many honors he was the recipient last year of the American Society of Agronomy's award for international service in agronomy.

JEAN MAYER ("The Dimensions of Human Hunger") is the new president of Tufts University. Before taking office in July he was professor of nutrition at Harvard University. Born and educated in Paris, Mayer served with distinction in both the French Army and the Free French forces during World War II. After the war he resumed his studies at Yale University, where in 1948 he received a Ph.D. in physiological chemistry. Two years later he was awarded his second doctorate (in physiology) by the

Sorbonne. He joined the Harvard faculty soon afterward. An expert on the problem of human obesity and the mechanism by which the body regulates its food intake, he has published some 650 papers and several books (the latest of which, *A Diet for Living,* appeared in 1975). Over the years he has served as a consultant to several United Nations agencies, including the Food and Agriculture Organization and the World Health Organization; at present he heads the UN Task Force on Child Nutrition. As chairman of the National Council on Hunger and Malnutrition in the U.S., he played a major role in calling the nation's attention to the nutritional problems of the poor in America. In 1969, as a special consultant to the President, he directed the First White House Conference on Food, Nutrition and Health. He has since served as chairman of the nutrition division of the White House Conference on the Aging, and he currently heads the health committee of the President's Consumer Advisory Council.

NEVIN S. SCRIMSHAW and VERNON R. YOUNG ("The Requirements of Human Nutrition") are members of the Department of Nutrition and Food Science at the Massachusetts Institute of Technology. Scrimshaw, who holds the rank of Institute Professor at M.I.T., has been head of the department since 1961; before that he served for 12 years as director of the Institute of Nutrition of Central America and Panama (IN-CAP). A graduate of Ohio Wesleyan University, he has three advanced degrees from Harvard University: an M.A. in biology (1939), a Ph.D. in physiology (1941) and an M.A. in public health (1959); he also holds an M.D. from the University of Rochester School of Medicine and Dentistry (1945). He continues to serve as a consultant to INCAP and travels frequently to Asia to advise on nutrition and health problems there. In addition he is a mem-

ber of a variety of advisory committees to Government departments, international agencies and private foundations. Among his present posts he is chairman of the World Health Organization's Advisory Committee on Medical Research, chairman of the International Nutrition Programs Committee of the National Research Council's Food and Nutrition Board and first vice-president of the International Union of Nutrition Sciences. Young, who is associate professor of nutritional biochemistry at M.I.T., was born in Wales and received his bachelor's degree in agriculture from the University of Reading. His Ph.D., in nutrition, is from the University of California at Davis. Since joining the faculty at M.I.T. in 1965 his research has tended to concentrate on the effects of old age on nutrient requirements and on the question of how lifelong nutrition might influence the rate at which the body ages.

JULES JANICK, CARL H. NOLLER and CHARLES L. RHYKERD ("The Cycles of Plant and Animal Nutrition") are on the faculty of Purdue University's School of Agriculture. Janick, who received his Ph.D. from Purdue in 1954, is a professor in the horticulture department. A specialist in the area of plant genetics and breeding (chiefly fruits), he is the editor of two professional journals (*HortScience* and the *Journal of the American Society for Horticultural Science*), author or coauthor of two textbooks (*Horticultural Science* and *Plant Science: An Introduction to World Crops*) and coeditor of two SCIENTIFIC AMERICAN readers (*Plant Agriculture* and *Food*). Noller, whose Ph.D. is from Michigan State University, is professor of animal sciences at Purdue. He teaches various courses in animal nutrition, with a research specialty in ruminant nutrition. Much of his research has been in collaboration with Rhykerd on the soil-plant-animal complex. Rhykerd, a 1957 Purdue Ph.D., started out as an assistant plant breeder for the De-Kalb Agricultural Association and Producers Seed Company and later became a soil scientist at the U.S. Pasture Laboratory in Pennsylvania. Since 1960 he has been a member of Purdue's agronomy department, where he now holds the rank of professor, working as a teacher and investigator in crop physiology and plant nutrition.

JACK R. HARLAN ("The Plants and Animals That Nourish Man") is professor of plant genetics in the crop-evolution laboratory of the department of agronomy of the University of Illinois at Urbana-Champaign. He was graduated from George Washington University in 1938 and received his Ph.D. in genetics from the University of California at Berkeley in 1942. For a number of years he worked as an agronomist for the U.S. Department of Agriculture. He later moved to Oklahoma, where he did research at the agricultural experimental station of the University of Oklahoma and taught at Oklahoma State University. He has been a member of the Illinois faculty since 1968. He is a past president of the Crop Science Society of America.

ROBERT S. LOOMIS ("Agricultural Systems") is professor in the department of agronomy and range science at the University of California at Davis. As an undergraduate at Iowa State University he majored in physics and minored in botany. Deciding to try for a career in quantitative botany, he went on to earn his M.S. from the University of Wisconsin for his work on the quantum efficiency of photosynthesis. He then spent two years in the Air Force, studying atmospheric physics at the Air Force Cambridge Research Center. After that, he writes, "my wife and I returned to Iowa for a season's work on her father's farm, where I coped with milking, haying and feeding hogs, and became convinced that crop physiology and agriculture were the way to go." He went back to Wisconsin to continue his study of botany and obtained a Ph.D. in 1956. In recent years, he reports, he and his colleagues at Davis have concentrated on the development of computer-simulated models of plant growth. Loomis was the first chairman of the ecology graduate group at Davis and served for three years as the director of the university's Institute of Ecology.

EARL O. HEADY ("The Agriculture of the U.S.") is Curtiss Distinguished Professor at Iowa State University, where he also directs the Center for Agricultural and Rural Development. Heady was born and raised on a farm in Nebraska and attended the University of Nebraska, where he acquired his B.Sc. and M.Sc. degrees. His doctorate is from Iowa State. A prolific researcher and writer, he has authored or coau-thored 17 books and more than 725 journal articles, research bulletins and monographs. He currently serves as vice-president of both the American Association of Agricultural Economists and the Canadian Agricultural Economics Association; he is also permanent chairman of the East-West Seminars for Agricultural Economists. In addition to his varied activities as a teacher, investigator and adviser on agricultural economics in the U.S., he notes, "I do a lot of work in developing countries, consulting with planners, evaluating policies for economic and agricultural development and analyzing development in general."

EDWIN J. WELLHAUSEN ("The Agriculture of Mexico") has played a key role in promoting the "green revolution" in Mexico as one of the leading agricultural investigators, teachers and administrators in that country for more than three decades. Before his retirement five years ago he served successively as head of the Rockefeller Foundation's corn-breeding program in Mexico from 1943 to 1952, director of the foundation's overall agricultural program in Mexico from 1952 to 1959, director of its International Corn Improvement Program from 1959 to 1963 and director general of the International Maize and Wheat Improvement Center from 1963 to 1971. A native of Oklahoma, he was educated at the University of Idaho, where he received a B.S. in plant pathology and agronomy in 1932, and at Iowa State University, where he obtained a Ph.D. in plant genetics in 1936. He taught and did research for several years at universities in the U.S. before joining the staff of the Rockefeller Foundation and moving to Mexico. Among his many contributions toward helping Mexico to reach self-sufficiency in food production, he has participated in the development of some 50 high-yielding hybrids and improved varieties of corn. In retirement he has continued his association with the Rockefeller Foundation as a special staff member. He writes: "My wife (a Colombian citizen) and I have our home in Mexico City, but it seems we are spending most of our time in other places in Latin America, with special emphasis on improving the production and general welfare of the traditional and subsistence farmers."

JOHN W. MELLOR ("The Agriculture of India") is chief economist of the Agency for International Development (AID) of the Department of State; he is on leave from his position as professor in the department of agricultural economics at Cornell University, where he directed the Program on Comparative Economic Development. His degrees are from Cornell (B.Sc., 1950; M.Sc., 1951; Ph.D., 1954) and the University of Oxford (diploma in agricultural economics, 1952). He has long had a special interest in India, having lived there on and off for a total of five years and having visited at least once a year since 1958. His most recent book, *The New Economics of Growth: A Strategy for India and the Developing World,* sets forth an overall development strategy based on vigorous growth in agriculture. Before joining AID he did consulting work for the Rockefeller Foundation, the World Bank, the Food and Agriculture Organization and other international development agencies; he continues to serve as vice-chairman of International Voluntary Services, a private predecessor of the Peace Corps. His primary professional concern now, he says, is "the relation between the national objectives and foreign-assistance program of the U.S. and the development strategies of the Third World."

ROGER REVELLE ("The Resources Available for Agriculture") is a professor at Harvard University, where he directs the Center for Population Studies. Before joining the Harvard faculty in 1964, he was associated for many years with the University of California, where he obtained his Ph.D. in 1936. He joined the staff of the university's Scripps Institution of Oceanography in 1931 as a research assistant and rose to become its director in 1951. From 1958 to 1961 he was also director of the university's campus at La Jolla and dean of the school of science and engineering. In 1961 he was appointed the first science adviser to the Secretary of the Interior, and when he returned to California in 1963, he became dean of research for all campuses. A wide-ranging investigator whose research interests over the years have included such diverse topics as the geology of the ocean floor, the analysis of the water resources of Pakistan and the demographic trends of the developing world, Revelle has been a frequent contributor to the pages of Scientific American.

PETER R. JENNINGS ("The Amplification of Agricultural Production") has contributed significantly to the amplification of world food production in his own career with the Rockefeller Foundation as a breeder of improved rice varieties. A graduate of Drew University, he joined the foundation in 1957, shortly after receiving his Ph.D. from Purdue University. His assignments since then have taken him to Colombia, where he served as director of the national rice program for the Ministry of Agriculture from 1957 to 1961, to the Philippines, where he headed the department of varietal improvement at the International Rice Research Institute from 1961 to 1967, and back to Colombia, where he supervised the rice-breeding program at the International Center of Tropical Agriculture from 1967 to 1975. He now works at the New York offices of the foundation as associate director for agricultural sciences.

W. DAVID HOPPER ("The Development of Agriculture in Developing Countries") is president of the International Development Research Centre in Ottawa. Before returning to his native country of Canada to take up his present job in 1970 he had lived for most of the previous decade in New Delhi, where he served first as the director of evaluation of the Ford Foundation's Intensive Agricultural Districts Program and later as associate field director of the Rocke-feller Foundation's Indian Agricultural Program and as visiting professor of agricultural economics at the Indian Agricultural Research Institute. A graduate of McGill University, he first went to India for an extended stay in 1953, when he received a Social Science Research Council fellowship to study the economic organization of a village on the Gangetic Plain in north-central India. He left India two years later to continue his graduate studies at Cornell University, where he obtained a Ph.D. in agricultural economics and cultural anthropology in 1957. After teaching for a time in Canada and the U.S. he went back to India in 1962 under the auspices of the Ford Foundation. During the latter half of the 1960's he was an important figure in the green revolution in Asian food production, working with the World Bank, the Asian Development Bank, the Food and Agriculture Organization, the major bilateral donor agencies and Asian governments to match the needs of programs to expand food production with internal and external sources of investment and assistance. He is currently chairman of the subcommittee of the Consultative Group for International Agricultural Research for the establishment of an International Centre for Agricultural Research in Dry Areas.

Bibliographies

Readers interested in further reading on the subjects covered by articles in this issue may find the lists below helpful.

FOOD AND AGRICULTURE

TRANSFORMING TRADITIONAL AGRICULTURE. Theodore W. Schultz. Yale University Press, 1964.

THE WORLD FOOD PROBLEM: A REPORT OF THE PRESIDENT'S SCIENCE ADVISORY COMMITTEE. May, 1967.

OVERCOMING WORLD HUNGER. Edited by Clifford M. Hardin. Prentice-Hall, Inc., 1969.

SUBSISTENCE AGRICULTURE AND ECONOMIC DEVELOPMENT. Edited by Clifton R. Wharton, Jr. Aldine Publishing Company, 1969.

BY BREAD ALONE. Lester R. Brown with Erik P. Eckholm. Praeger Publishers, 1974.

A RICHER HARVEST: NEW HORIZONS FOR DEVELOPING COUNTRIES. Sudhir Sen. Orbis Books, 1974.

MEETING FOOD NEEDS IN THE DEVELOPING WORLD: THE LOCATION AND MAGNITUDE OF THE TASK IN THE NEXT DECADE. International Food Policy Research Institute, February, 1976.

THE DIMENSIONS OF HUMAN HUNGER

FOOD AND POPULATION: THE WRONG PROBLEM? Jean Mayer in *Daedalus,* Vol. 93, No. 3, pages 830–844; Summer, 1964.

THE NUTRITION FACTOR: ITS ROLE IN DEVELOPMENT. Alan Berg. Brookings Institution, 1973.

NUTRITION. *Science,* Vol. 188, No. 4188, pages 557–577; May 9, 1975.

THE WORLD FOOD PROSPECT. Lester R. Brown in *Science,* Vol. 190, No. 4219, pages 1053–1059; December 12, 1975.

THE REQUIREMENTS OF HUMAN NUTRITION

RECOMMENDED DIETARY ALLOWANCES. Food and Nutrition Board, National Research Council. National Academy of Sciences, 1974.

DIETARY STANDARDS. D. Mark Hegsted in *Journal of the American Dietetic Association,* Vol. 66, No. 1, pages 13–21; January, 1976.

SHATTUCK LECTURE—STRENGTHS AND WEAKNESSES OF THE COMMITTEE APPROACH: AN ANALYSIS OF PAST AND PRESENT RECOMMENDED DIETARY ALLOWANCES FOR PROTEIN IN HEALTH AND DISEASE. Nevin S. Scrimshaw in *The New England Journal of Medicine,* Vol. 294, No. 3, pages 136–142, January 15, 1976; No. 4, pages 198–203, January 22, 1976.

THE CYCLES OF PLANT AND ANIMAL NUTRITION

THE NATURE AND PROPERTIES OF SOILS. Harry O. Buckman and Nyle C. Brady. The Macmillan Company, 1960.

ENERGY EXCHANGE IN THE BIOSPHERE. David M. Gates. Harper & Row, Publishers, 1962.

ANIMAL NUTRITION. Leonard A. Maynard and John K. Loosli. McGraw-Hill Book Company, Inc., 1969.

NUTRIENT REQUIREMENTS OF DOMESTIC ANIMALS: NUTRIENT REQUIREMENTS OF BEEF CATTLE (1970), DAIRY CATTLE (1971), POULTRY (1971), SWINE (1973), SHEEP (1975). National Academy of Sciences.

AGRICULTURAL PRODUCTION AND ENERGY RESOURCES. G. H. Heichel in *American Scientist,* Vol. 64, No. 1, pages 64–72; January–February, 1976.

THE PLANTS AND ANIMALS THAT NOURISH MAN

THE DOMESTICATION AND EXPLOITATION OF PLANTS AND ANIMALS. Edited by P. J. Ucko and D. W. Dimbleby. Aldine Publishing Company, 1969.

PALAEOETHNOBOTANY: THE PREHISTORIC FOOD PLANTS OF THE NEAR EAST AND EUROPE. Jane M. Renfrew. Columbia University Press, 1973.

CROPS & MAN. Jack R. Harlan. American Society of Agronomy, 1975.

AGRICULTURAL SYSTEMS

FARMING SYSTEMS OF THE WORLD. A. N. Duckham and G. B. Masefield. Chatto & Windus, 1971.

THE AGRICULTURAL SYSTEMS OF THE WORLD: AN EVOLUTIONARY APPROACH. D. B. Grigg. Cambridge University Press, 1974.

ANIMAL AGRICULTURE: THE BIOLOGY OF DOMESTIC ANIMALS AND THEIR USE BY MAN. Edited by H. H. Cole and Magnar Ronning. W. H. Freeman and Company, 1974.

PRINCIPLES OF FIELD CROP PRODUCTION. John H. Martin, Warren H. Leonard and David L. Stamp. Macmillan Publishing Co., Inc., 1976.

THE AGRICULTURE OF THE U.S.

AGRICULTURAL POLICY UNDER ECONOMIC DEVELOPMENT. Earl O. Heady. Iowa State University Press, 1962.

A PRIMER ON FOOD, AGRICULTURE, AND PUBLIC POLICY. Earl O. Heady. Random House, 1967.

FOUNDATIONS OF FARM POLICY. Luther Tweeten. University of Nebraska Press, 1970.

THE AGRICULTURE OF MEXICO

ROCKEFELLER FOUNDATION COLLABORATION IN AGRICULTURAL RESEARCH IN MEXICO. E. J. Wellhausen in *Agronomy Journal,* Vol. 42, No. 4, pages 167–175; April, 1950.

STRATEGIES FOR INCREASING AGRICULTURAL PRODUCTION ON SMALL HOLDINGS. Centro Internacional de Mejoramiento de Maíz y Trigo, 1970.

SEVEN YEARS OF EXPERIENCE: 1967–1973. Centro Internacional de Mejoramiento de Maíz y Trigo, 1974.

THE AGRICULTURE OF INDIA

THE WONDER THAT WAS INDIA. A. L. Basham. Sidgwick and Jackson, 1954.

AGRICULTURAL TRENDS IN INDIA, 1891–1947: OUTPUT, WELFARE, AND PRODUCTIVITY. George Blyn. University of Pennsylvania Press, 1961.

THE ECONOMICS OF AGRICULTURAL DEVELOPMENT. John W. Mellor. Cornell University Press, 1966.

DEVELOPING RURAL INDIA: PLAN AND PRACTICE. Edited by John W. Mellor, Thomas F. Weaver, Uma J. Lele and Sheldon R. Simon. Cornell University Press, 1968.

FOOD GRAIN MARKETING IN INDIA. Uma J. Lele. Cornell University Press, 1971.

THE DESIGN OF RURAL DEVELOPMENT: LESSONS FROM AFRICA. Uma Lele. The Johns Hopkins University Press, 1975.

THE RESOURCES AVAILABLE FOR AGRICULTURE

FOOD FROM THE LAND. Sterling B. Hendricks in *Resources and Man: A Study and Recommendations.* Committee on Resources and Man of the Division of Earth Sciences, National Academy of Sciences–National Research Council. W. H. Freeman and Company, 1969.

FOOD FROM THE SEA. William E. Ricker in *Resources and Man: A Study and Recommendations.* Committee on Resources and Man of the Division of Earth Sciences, National Academy of Sciences–National Research Council. W. H. Freeman and Company, 1969.

ENERGY USE IN THE U.S. FOOD SYSTEM. John S. Steinhart and Carol E. Steinhart in *Science,* Vol. 184, No. 4134, pages 307–316; April 19, 1974.

ENERGY AND LAND CONSTRAINTS IN FOOD PROTEIN PRODUCTION. David Pimentel, William Dritschilo, John Krummel and John Kutzman in *Science,* Vol. 190, No. 4216, pages 754–761; November 21, 1975.

WILL THE EARTH'S LAND AND WATER RESOURCES BE SUFFICIENT FOR FUTURE POPULATIONS? Roger Revelle in *Report of the Symposium on Population, Resources and the Environment (Stockholm 26 September–5 October, 1973).* United Nations, 1973.

ENERGY USE IN RURAL INDIA. Roger Revelle in *Science,* Vol. 192, No. 4243, pages 969–975; June 4, 1976.

THE AMPLIFICATION OF AGRICULTURAL PRODUCTION

RICE BREEDING AND WORLD FOOD PRODUCTION. Peter R. Jennings in *Science,* Vol. 186, No. 4169, pages 1085–1088; December 20, 1974.

THE WORLD FOOD SITUATION: A NEW INITIATIVE. Sterling Wortman. The Rockefeller Foundation; December, 1975.

STRATEGY FOR THE ALLEVIATION OF WORLD HUNGER. Sterling Wortman. The Rockefeller Foundation, 1976.

THE WORLD FOOD SITUATION AND TECHNICAL ASSISTANCE. Sterling Wortman. The Rockefeller Foundation, 1976.

THE IMPACT OF HIGH-YIELDING RICE VARIETIES IN LATIN AMERICA WITH SPECIAL EMPHASIS ON COLOMBIA: A PRELIMINARY REPORT. Grant M. Scobie and Rafael Posada. Centro Internacional de Agricultura Tropical; April, 1976.

FOOD CROPS IN THE LOW-INCOME COUNTRIES: THE STATE OF PRESENT AND EXPECTED AGRICULTURAL RESEARCH AND TECHNOLOGY. Ralph W. Cummings, Jr. The Rockefeller Foundation; May, 1976.

THE DEVELOPMENT OF AGRICULTURE IN DEVELOPING COUNTRIES

GETTING AGRICULTURE MOVING: ESSENTIALS FOR DEVELOPMENT AND MODERNIZATION. Arthur T. Mosher. Frederick A. Praeger, Publishers, 1966.

ASIAN AGRICULTURAL SURVEY. Asian Development Bank. Tokyo University Press, 1969.

Index

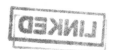

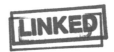